LONGEVITY TRAINING

"ANTI-AGE COACH, LIFESTYLE ANALYSIS, BREATHING, POSTURE, NUTRITION, SKINCARE, TOP SECRETS TO LONG LIFE AND STAYING YOUNG"

WRITTEN BY STEVE CHEN

TABLE OF CONTENTS

INTRODUCTION

Living a long time does not necessarily mean living well and longevity does not automatically translate into quality of life. How satisfying is it to live a long time without truly living to your fullest abilities and capabilities?

Longevity is best experienced in a context that includes the best health characteristics: energy, vitality, physical strength and primary strength. And beyond those dimensions of health, there are others that illuminate well-being: positive moods, self-confidence, cognitive clarity, creativity, and self-realization. Even more, there are states of being that are called transcendent, which belong to the highest levels of self-expression. The transcendent states are the road to a healthier mental strength.

All these aspects of health are related and intertwined, interrelated and interactive. Improvement everywhere has a chain effect everywhere. Often, improving only one aspect of oneself has beneficial repercussions on the whole being.

Longevity training seeks the most efficient ways to expand global well-being, opening the limits of life. The training focuses on the essential factors that determine longevity, from the improvement of the fundamental mechanics of the body to the recruitment of the dynamic forces of the mind.

CHAPTER ONE

LONGEVITY TRAINING

Longevity is defined as a term that commonly refers to "long life" or "enormous duration of life." The word "longevity" is sometimes used as a synonym for "life expectancy" in demography. Several factors contribute to the longevity of an individual. Even among those who do not desire eternal life, one could desire the longevity of experiencing more than life or making a greater contribution to humanity. It can help make medicine for longevity and a longer and healthier life a reality.

Current research on aging and longevity shows that life expectancy is now 74 and 80 years and could be significantly longer with the anti-aging advances that are currently being investigated. This research suggests a promising way to find and develop medications to prolong life and prevent or treat aging-related diseases. These ideas could shed light on human aging since it is known that humans and some bacteria have mutually beneficial relationships. The idea behind the dividend on longevity was clearly expressed in a book by the scientist that claimed that the research should have had the direct objective of delaying the seven-year aging process. The researchers were also interested in the influence of healthy and less healthy foods on mortality.

THE BASICS OF LONGEVITY

The secrets of longevity are the basis for living a healthy and harmonious lifestyle and existence. With degenerative diseases so rampant in our societies with cancer and cardiovascular diseases at the top of the list, it is necessary to return to the basics. Creating a fundamental basis for achieving and maintaining a healthy existence should be our first objective.

To achieve this basic basis, we must continually focus our attention on certain areas that shape our physical, mental, and emotional development. Three important aspects that require our attention are nutrition, exercise, and stress reduction. When we can master these three areas of self-development, we can live a longer and healthier life.

NUTRITION: Nutrition is important to live a healthy and long life, because what we eat matters. The food we put in the mouth is digested and used as nutrients for cell development and survival. Many people lack proper nutrition to nourish their body cells. Because cells lack adequate nutrition, a person can resort to overeating. Unfortunately, overfeeding does not lead to better nutrition. In general, incorrect substances are obtained, which negatively affect our level of health.

Eating well consists of eating many fruits and vegetables since these food sources have the highest amount of nutrients. If you need to eat meat to get your daily protein intake, focus on lean meats such as fresh and salty fish and other poultry meat. Stay away from unhealthy meat like red meat.

In addition to eating well, you must fill your body with plenty of water, since H2O is one of the most vital nutrients on the planet. The human body is composed of 70 to 75 percent water and the human brain composed more than 95 percent water. Getting your body rehydrated is essential for your health and longevity.

The exercise is important since the human body was designed by God, Nature or the Universe to move. The movement is part of our existence. To do anything, we must have a realm of uninhibited and unlocked movement. However, when we do not get the exercise that the body requires to remain flexible and agile, it oxidizes. The body does not need intense exercise to get a good workout.

Walking is an excellent form of exercise. If you walk during the day for 20-30 minutes, you can exercise daily and the vital nutrients that sunlight provides to humans. Other forms of exercise that keep the body full of energy and vitality include yoga, qigong, tai chi, and pilates. For yoga and pilates, you should focus on delicate styles that tone your muscles and test your level of flexibility and strength.

STRESS REDUCTION: Stress reduction is important for a healthy lifestyle because too much stress leads to mental and physical illness. Having a little stress in life is fine, but it should be balanced and eliminated whenever possible. Enduring too much stress for too long can make a person physically ill. Stress drains a person's energy, hinders cell communication, and forms nodes in the muscles of the body through tension.

Some forms of stress reduction include breathing, meditation, and exercise. Walking again is excellent for human health because it causes the body to move, pump blood, and reduce stress.

If you can concentrate on these three basic lifestyle options (nutrition, exercise, and stress reduction), you can establish a longevity basis.

THE BEST EXERCISE ROUTINE FOR LONGEVITY

Walk fast for an hour every day.

It doesn't have to happen suddenly. For instance, if the train station is a 15-minute walk from your home and you do it anyway, it's 30 minutes there. Therefore, you can choose a cafeteria 15 minutes walk from your office and make a daily visit. These may not be your exact circumstances, but an idea is made: find places that can be explored on foot and go there every day. On weekends, ensure you walk everywhere you go, even in faraway places: do your best to leave your car in the garage or at the entrance of your home throughout the weekend.

Cardiovascular exercise for 2.5 to 5 hours per week

Running, biking or swimming are good options, but the type of exercise you choose is not important. The key is to work your body to the point of breathing quickly and sweating. A simple way to reach this threshold is to have a stationary bike and a road bike (to leave when the weather permits, otherwise go home) and take a 30 to 40-minute walk every two days and a total of 2 hours at the end of the week

Use weight exercises or weightless exercises to strengthen all muscles.

This may be the classic routine in the gym, but your muscles get stronger when you climb the stairs instead of the elevator (Longo advises you to climb the stairs always!), Walk instead of driving, grow food in your garden instead of buying them, and do manual work at home instead of hiring someone to do it. When participating in a weight training session, consume at least 30 grams of protein in a single meal within 1-2 hours to maximize muscle growth.

In terms of weekly runtime, research shows that most of the beneficial effects are caused by the first 2.5 hours. For example, a study conducted in Australia which had more than 200,000 respondents, aged 45 to 75 found that those who exercised (at moderate or vigorous levels) at least 2.5 hours a week had a 47% reduction in overall mortality. The increase of 5 hours per week led to a 54% reduction in mortality. Ensuring that at least part of this activity is in the vigorous range has reduced the risk of death by 12 percentage.

Another extensive study involving more than 650,000 people in the United States and Europe has shown that mortality has been reduced by 31% for people who have practiced at least 2.5 hours a week with moderate intensity (or more than 75 minutes at vigorous intensity). The increase in total exercise at 5 hours at moderate intensity (or 2.5 hours at vigorous levels) reduced the risk of death by 37%.

Examples of physical activity you can practice include walking fast or jogging slowly (faster than 4 mph), biking (10-12 mph) or gardening. Examples of strenuous physical activity involve climbing stairs or walking, cycling (more than 12 mph), playing soccer or jogging (more than 4 mph).

Therefore, there is undoubtedly an additional benefit of going up to 4 hours of training a week, with some of the exercises and training. There might be diminishing returns after 2.5 hours and you want to avoid overloading your body by going beyond the weekly limit of 5 hours. Excessive exercise causes damage to the knees, hips and joints over time. You do not want your body to break prematurely due to excessive exercises.

ENERGY PRODUCTION

A key ingredient for longevity is energy. Energy feeds all organ systems, including the heart and the brain. Body energy production and how its production can be fully maximized will be discussed at this point.

The primary source of all biochemical energy comes from nutrients. The nutrients in food are decomposed or broken down by metabolism from higher to a lower energy level. As a result, energy is accumulated for personal use. Without energy we can not move our bodies, nor would we be able to think correctly and create thoughts.

What type of nutrients provides the body with optimal energy? The science behind longevity is interested in advanced nutrient selection. However, high energy metabolism also depends on the logical use of the numerous cofactors that are relevant to the dynamics of metabolism: enzymes, minerals, vitamins and, where appropriate, nutrients derived from botanical substances and new molecules discovered through new medical research and analysis.

The body energy production depends on the adequate functioning of mitochondria, and the subcellular organelles specialized in the extraction of energy from nutrients. Cell types differ in their mitochondrial content. For example, the heart, which needs constant vigor, has cells that contain several thousand mitochondria each; Skin cells, on the other hand, can function with a few dozen. Brain cells are also energy intensive. Each organ has specific types of mitochondrial populations with unique and different requirements. Longevity training implements the new science of biological energy to expand the life span and quality of life.

THE INTERIOR TERRITORY

The experience of our inner landscape leaps more vividly into consciousness once the eyes are closed. The territory of the internal body is an image painted by the signals that enter the consciousness from the totality of all sensory units.

Internal awareness provides not only a perception of incoming body signals but also a channel for the mind to send healing signals to the body. This forms the basis for communication techniques with internal organ systems. These techniques include self-guided relaxation, dynamic imaging, self-hypnosis, autogenic training and meditation.

Stress: It can be said that the nerve centers of the body and the old emotional circuits of the brain have their own minds. In fact, they can react robotically to life events, often not only to our disgust but could also affect our lives. Cardiac reactivity, for instance, describes a tendency to respond to life events with increases in heart rate and blood pressure. The same can be said of excessive intestinal, respiratory, muscular and cutaneous activity.

Excessive activity of the organs is not only unnecessary, but it is also harmful to the body and, if chronic, can cause anatomical lesions. Stress can cause a spectrum of symptoms such as fatigue, headaches, sleep disorders, anxiety and depression. Stress reduces lifespan.

Longevity training attempts to convert stress reactions into positive physical and mental energies.

Organ health: Longevity training refers to the proper functioning of all organ systems so that each organ lives vigorously and all organs live in harmony. Organ systems include cardiovascular, gastrointestinal, respiratory, skeletal-muscular, hematological, immune, endocrine, neurological and special organs. The health and harmony of organ systems are fundamental to longevity.

The body is efficient in terms of longevity if it is maintained within a certain weight range. Lungs do not like smoking more or arteries, and only a small part of the brain appreciates smoking. Longevity training tries to change habit patterns to reduce and then eliminate damage.

The body responds to physical exercise. Exercise massages all internal organs. The glands are stimulated, the bones receive signs of strengthening, the heart is trained to beat more solidly and gain resistance. However, aerobic exercise, while improving longevity, must be judiciously measured according to one's abilities. Aerobic exercise too small and too excessive, both work against longevity.

Several non-aerobic exercise disciplines develop full body-mind connections. They involve the use of guided meditative consciousness to flow progressively in neuromuscular networks. Longevity training makes important use of this type of meditation.

Sleep health is important for longevity. Balancing circadian rhythms, creating relaxation in dreams and stimulating the regeneration of sleep patterns to promote well-being and optimal productivity during the day.

OBJECTIVES OF EFFECTIVE LONGEVITY TRAINING FOR LONGER LIFE SPAN

As the body strengthens, the mind also strengthens and this forces the mind to master new patterns of experience that conserve energy and activate health.

Through special techniques adapted individually, the mind is trained to create special states of consciousness that give vitality to the networks of the body.

What experiences are sought in these special states of consciousness? Although each person may report differently, a comforting sense of tranquillity, a relaxing experience of detachment and a greater perception of physical strength and personal power are often expressed. Many people often admit that they experience pleasant feelings, have a peaceful state of mind and become happy when they are at home. Words often do not adequately describe these special states.

The neural basis of the power of mental images: The images, as used in longevity training, involve the conscious creation of mental representations that may contain visual images such as scenarios of dreams, sounds, words and phrases that are rhythmically pleasing and, above all, pleasant feelings and primary emotions.

Mental images derive from consciously activated brain areas. Neurons from different parts of the brain are well represented in the images used, each corresponding to extensive neural networks. The more diverse the images, the greater the areas of the brain that act and the more effective the therapeutic impact is when the waves of the neural networks resonate at the edges of the nervous system.

Healing images in longevity training must be individually adapted to respect the preferences of conscious and unconscious minds. Each practice reinforces healing images, expanding its systemic reach, working on reprogramming the neural substrate of the mind permanently.

MEDITATION

Meditation incorporates a set of techniques that use consciousness as a vehicle to expand human awareness in bodily territories and create an increase in consciousness itself.

The mental states briefly described above are the doors to other states that are called transcendent. There is a great need for the scientific study of transcendent states because they represent the penultimate connectivity of body and mind.

There are various types of techniques for meditation and it is crucial to select one that suits one's preferences and talents. The preferred techniques should be fun.

Self-hypnosis: Although the special mental states achieved through meditation and self-hypnosis share common characteristics, the process of techniques differs. Self-hypnosis is based on the ability to induce a hypnotic state on its own, usually using a series of reflexes learned. Once the hypnotic state is reached, the response to mental images increases. As a result, personal changes can take place more quickly.

Longevity training is based on the mind's potential to exceed its usual functioning astronomically. By crossing their routine boundaries, the mind can be guided to reach more richness of its dimensions.

Longevity training also seeks to expand the power of the body by appreciating its dynamics from the infinitely small, such as chromosomes, mitochondria, and cellular metabolism, to large, as in organ systems.

Concerning the body and the mind, ultimately there are no limits that separate the two; everything is a continuum. Longevity training respects this vision of life and health.

ANTI-AGING BENEFITS OF STRENGTH TRAINING

Research from Penn State Medical College, the University of Sydney and Columbia University has established that regular strength training has important benefits for longevity.

Natural displacement is an integral part of the lifestyle of blue areas. Most of the centurions did not belong to gyms; they ran marathons or iron bombs. Instead, natural movements such as walking to work and climbing stairs and working muscles doing manual labor, such as gardening and housework, have been integrated into your daily life. Unfortunately, for most of us, the natural movement was designed for our lives. Marilynn Preston's next advice has some good ideas for those who want to start doing some.

Physical exercise: There are many beneficial reasons for strength training beyond just looking good in skinny outfits. Strong bodies are connected to strong minds. Strength training creates confidence, healthy muscles and tissues. It is also good for stable joints, injury prevention and weight loss. However, despite that, there are less than 25 percent of Americans over 45 years of age who work with weights or practice strength training regularly. Much less, I imagine.

 Blame our sedentary lifestyles. The heaviest thing that many of us raise is our laptop. Nothing we do requires that we raise our arms above our heads. So, for all those reasons and more, here are eight truths about strength training to consider, as you decide how and when to start:

There are no age limits: Young children have to wait for their bodies and bones to be strong enough to withstand the stress of weight training, but the rest of us can start where we are and expect to see significant improvements over time. The body is magnificent in this way. 90-year-olds are pumping iron and getting stronger, and so are you, once you understand the basics.

Technique is everything: This is an important problem because if you do not learn to rise consciously, aware of your breathing, posture, core and limitations, you can tense a muscle or tear a tendon. Find an evolved teacher/coach or taught by books or videos online.

Lift heavier weights: It will not be strengthened by lifting the same weight of five or ten pounds day after day. However, for your muscles to become strengthened, you must challenge them, gradually, over time, with heavier weights. The amount of "correct" weight will always vary, but this principle remains the same: you should be able to do a dozen repetitions correctly, with the last two a real fight.

Inside or outside the gym: Both will build strength. The use of machines in the gym generally has a price. Free weights speak for themselves: always and everywhere. The devices used in gym have a limited range of motion; Free weights have endless benefits. Both can work if you apply intensive, consistent, careful, and proper attention to your breathing method. Exercises with body weight (squats, push-ups, lunges) should also be part of your routine, so it is smart to consult someone who has experience at the beginning. By the way, lifting body weight in yoga also increases strength!

Expect pain: It is known as DOMS (delayed onset muscle soreness) and that's what you should expect after a great workout session. Pain is a different feeling "No pain, no gain" is not a way to approach a sustainable strength training practice. If your coach thinks otherwise, look for another coach who understands better.

Know your body: Spend some time looking at anatomical drawings to learn about the kidneys of the colon, the patella of the pubic bone. Developing a better body awareness will help you create and perform a balanced workout: from front to back, from side to side, pushing and pulling, expanding and contracting.

Be efficient: A twenty minute workout can be as good as a forty minute workout if you know what you are doing and why you are doing it. Compound movements, for example, a bicep curl combined with a lunge, will give you twice the benefits in half the time. Therefore, it will be a super slow lift and high-intensity interval training. Again, study and experiment until you find a routine that gives you joy. If you can do it two or three times a week, over time, your body will change extraordinarily, unless you celebrate each workout with two cereal bars and three beers.

Use it or lose it: It is an uncomfortable truth that as we get older, we lose our muscles and weaken unless we make an effort to remain strong, flexible, agile and juicy. It's about working with what you have during the time you have and being grateful in the middle.

CHAPTER TWO

THE ROLE OF STRENGTH TRAINING

These studies laid the groundwork for the hypothesis that men in physically active jobs had a lower risk of heart disease than men in physically inactive jobs. Therefore, it has been proposed that a sedentary lifestyle increases the risk of heart disease.

Since then, it has been repeatedly shown that regular exercise is associated with a lower risk of premature death, coronary heart disease, certain types of cancer and diabetes. It has also been proven that exercise and physical activity improves mental health. The World Health Organization (WHO) has recently recognized physical inactivity as one of the leading global risk factors for premature morbidity and mortality.

However, there are still questions like what type of physical exercise is likely to improve your healthy lifestyle? Should we take a walk, jog, lift weights? And is there an easy way to evaluate or measure our physical conditions?

The physical form consists of the cardiorespiratory form and the muscular form. Aerobic exercises are recommended for the benefit of the heart, such as walking, jogging, swimming or cycling, and strength and stretching exercises for strength and flexibility in general.

However, strength training may have broader implications for general health than previously thought. Evidence suggests that muscle strength is inversely and independently associated with death from all causes after adapting to cardiorespiratory fitness and other cofactors such as age, body fat, smoking, alcohol, and hypertension.

MUSCLE STRENGTH AND LONGEVITY

In 2015, German researchers published a narrative review of studies that address the role of muscle strength as a predictor of mortality. Fourteen epidemiological studies met the study criteria and all reported that an increase in the level of muscle strength was significantly associated with lower mortality from all causes. The same model was observed for cardiovascular mortality. Existing studies have not shown that low muscle strength is predictive of cancer mortality.

Muscle strength and longevity: the role of strength training

Grip strength is a simple and economical measure of overall muscle strength. Grip strength is a economical and simple measure of overall muscle strength. It is usually done with a Jamar hydraulic dynamometer capable of measuring isometric grip strength with excellent reliability and reproducibility.

Is strength training associated with the benefits of mortality?

The connection between grip strength and mortality does not provide evidence that strength training improves health and longevity. Although the epidemiological data available are reliable, it cannot be said whether there is a causal relationship between muscle strength and mortality.

Randomized studies on the effects of strength training on mortality are difficult to perform. There would be a high risk of crossing between groups. Also, an in-depth study would be needed to confirm whether or not there is a benefit to mortality.

Possible mechanisms underlying the effects of strength training

There may be several reasons why strength training and grip strength are associated with longevity.

Resistance training can counteract the decrease in muscle mass and age-related strength (sarcopenia), which is characterized by a reduction in contractile proteins and an excessive accumulation of intra-and extracellular lipids.

Strength training also improves neuromuscular coordination and balance. This can reduce the risk of fall injuries that often provide serious threats to the health of the elderly.

Besides, resistance training increases bone mass and mineral density and reduces the risk of osteoporosis, which is a global public health problem.

It has been shown that skeletal muscle acts in many ways as an endocrine organ. Skeletal muscle cells produce cytokines (myokines) that can help fight inflammation and maintain normal body function. Therefore, myokine can contribute to exercise-induced protection against various chronic diseases. Strength training can also improve cardiovascular risk factors such as blood pressure, blood lipids and insulin resistance.

TRAINING IN LONGEVITY: CONSCIOUS FITNESS FOR THE MIND AND BODY

Longevity training is a conscious physical state of the body. It is an intentional training designed towards living a longer, healthier and happier life in a stronger, more flexible and balanced body. Instead of training to appease the ego standards of what we believe we should see based on what the media and society tell us, it is functional aptitude. Create and maintain the ability to carry out the activities we love to perform as easily as possible for as long as possible. What's the point of looking a certain way if we don't feel well? Wouldn't it be better to feel good, work well, look and be healthy? Exercises, which can be strength, flexibility, rehabilitation, yoga or pilates, kung fu, tai chi or qigong, are intuitively prescribed moment by moment depending on what the client needs and wants.

We are whole beings made of body, emotions and the mind. It is said that our body is like a living metaphor for the mind and emotions. When we accumulate stress, both mentally and emotionally, if not treated healthily, stress manifests itself in the body. Longevity training also addresses any problem that arises at the time to improve, heal and adapt as a whole so that we can achieve and experience everything we want. The body is an adaptive thing. It adapts to your environment. For this it was designed. It adapts to its surroundings and to what it perceives. He perceives what you think and what you believe. The human brain cannot tell the difference between what you see with your eyes and what you imagine in your mind. He feels that both are real. Therefore, it would be very useful if the thoughts you are thinking support what you want to experience.

FUNCTIONAL LONGEVITY EXERCISES

When it comes to increasing your physical function for a long time, which exercises are the best? Here are some of the best practical yet functional longevity exercises out there. Some common characteristics of high quality functional longevity exercises include:

Influence on energy systems for longevity: There are growing ways to manipulate and improve your health that will lead you to a healthier life. The more you practice them, the greater the cumulative effects on the outcome of your health. Our bodies are incredibly complex things that resist change of any kind. "Keeping things as they are" is one of the main functions of our body. Make changes; Spiritual, mentally, emotionally or physically requires the application of knowledge at many levels to achieve results.

Taking a well-chosen pill will probably give you the result you are looking for. However, there is no magic bullet. An adjustment will produce some limited results. The combination of many improvements will multiply the effect on longevity. Here we are also looking for an improvement in the quality of life. Practicing these improvements every day, without fail, will help you maintain the extension of your life, Longevity.

Internal energy systems: The following cosmic connections must be well built and consolidated. When they are not, all kinds of; Mental, emotional, physical and even spiritual problems may arise. Managing the right advice and metaphysical therapy is essential here.

The Higher Self: The opening of the *"higher self"* will connect the individual with a "greater creative" consciousness, the Great Love, the Unity of all Creation and the special part that we have to play in it. When this "Cosmic Connection" is established, the individual becomes deeply aware of the value of life, especially his. This experience changes lives and is challenging. Life acquires a new meaning and a new direction when you "know" who you are and where you are in the "scheme of things."

Once we have opened the Higher Self, we can explore other areas of our consciousness. We can unlock areas of; clairvoyance, clairvoyance, etc. Discovering our "superior skills" is not only rewarding but essential. It can help us grow beyond our limits, to give us more meaning and purpose in this life and more in our spiritual evolution.

The chakras: In general, by stimulating the upper Chakras, our spiritual, mental and emotional abilities will open. Stimulating our lower Chakras will improve our earthly activities. Care must be taken when stimulating these *"centers of power."* When an incorrect type of energy or too much energy is sent through these Vortices, the lower Systems (nerves, brain, etc.) can overload and "burn."

The general approach is to improve with balance. The individual stimulation of the Centres sometimes moves the condition only to another level, so it must be rebalanced. Testing, recording and completing a "combined balance treatment" is much more effective, since treating more Chakras together will give a better result by improving the whole. Getting the right knowledge and training here is essential, not only to properly stimulate but also to map what you want to explore and achieve.

Meridians: This simple but effective alternative healing system has been around for some time. It requires extensive training and practice. Chinese "barefoot doctors" have deeply used this healing system. They would travel from one city to another, making it an essential health service for the villages. Farmers who work hard on poor diets have found that this health service is essential to keep their bodies healthy and free from disturbance. This tradition has been transmitted to modern acupuncture and acupressure practices and remains a key addition to the healing options available to us.

We can improve the health and longevity of our bodies by stimulating these *"energy centers"* that are already within us. These "doors" in our true selves are waiting to be discovered and opened. There are many areas within us where we can "take advantage" and influence to give ourselves a longer, happier and healthier life. "Quality of life" is also important, because this is where we really begin to experience the true wonder that our body is in this life.

CHAPTER THREE

BRAIN STIMULATION FOR AGING, LONGEVITY AND PROSPEROUS LIFE

The power of the brain is enormous and if it is programmed in the right way, it is capable of achieving much more than what we do today. Mental programming is extremely essential to bring longevity to the human brain and to life in general. To understand mental programming, one must know that the mind exists in two states, conscious and subconscious.

The first state is when we are aware of our actions and do them voluntarily. Whereas in the subconscious state, we are not aware of our actions but we do them. This can also happen in a hypnotic mental state. These actions are responsible for the general character of a person and the way of life. To live a healthy life, it is necessary to program them well and increase the longevity of the brain.

The brain can be positively stimulated and scientists have shown that there are areas or points in the brain that, if really stimulated or used correctly, can lead to excellent results. There are tools/techniques that can capture the pulsations of the brain and the points given by the nerve cells of the mind.

Research that analyzed Albert Einstein's brain found that his brain was different from the others, in the sense that he had more interconnections between his neurons. Cerebral longevity is not based on the number of neurons but on the diversity of interconnections between neurons. It is interesting to note that interconnections are not inherited, but are created by the individual. When these interconnections are not used, they shrink and die but when they are constantly engaged in mental training, they tend to expand and strengthen.

This helps to expand the power of the mind into completely new dimensions of thought and experience. The whole concept of brain stimulation towards longevity derives from the use of a technology that supports the theory of mental programming and penetrates the subconscious mind and makes efforts to alter things in life, such as addictions, phobias and character defects.

Such mental programming exists in many different types, such as subliminal suggestions, affirmation speeches, meditation, yoga and aromatherapy, etc. But the latest trend that is catching up quickly is the capture of brain waves. This technique helps to synchronize brain waves in sync with the electrical impulses that are sent through audio signals from an external source.

Because brain waves are of many types, such as the alpha, beta, theta and gamma states, brain wave technology can be used to create several changes in thoughts and, therefore, improve the lifestyle of a person in a more positive way. Brain longevity can be improved by brain wave technology. The brain is the most crucial part of the human body and is a handy tool that, if used correctly, can produce miraculous results. More and more people are waking up to this fact and this is really a change for a better and better life.

Brain stimulation for longevity requires dealing with the physical form of the brain. Some people do not even listen to brain fitness because they believe that absolutely nothing can be done to improve brain function. They believed that the functioning of their brains is destined to diminish as they age. Brain stimulation for a longer life span is possible. The fact that the brain is not a muscle does not make its response to activity different. Like the muscles of the body, the greater use of the brain improves its functioning, while its underutilization only serves to deteriorate it. This explains why most of the innovations were the result of minds that worked day and night. The more the brain is involved, the more acute it becomes to counteract the pressure.

However, brain stimulation for longevity requires techniques slightly different from those used in physical form. This explains the development of brainwave entrainment technology that serves not only to improve mental power but also to prolong its period of functioning. There are many aspects improved by this technology that includes:

1. Learn and experience new things. Try out new and fascinating things to learn that you know very little about. Visiting the library for more information on the subject or finding information on the subject on the internet will stimulate your brain. After obtaining the information, behave as if you were an expert who informs others of what you have learned. Teach them how little you know about the subject. Then, look for another topic. This activates the mind in incredible ways. Also, You can use other brainwave equipment, such as CDs, that have been produced specially for learning purposes.

2. Watch educational programs on television. Television programs such as documentaries will make you discover things you ignored and increase your ability to reason. Try to analyze the characters in such documentaries. This will do a lot to stimulate your brain.

3. Play challenging games such as crosswords, card games, Sudoku and other similar games. Games of this type make you feel better because they require critical thinking to make you win.

With the development of brainwave entrainment technology, your mind can stay as fresh as ever while alive.

STIMULATE GROWTH HORMONE FOR LONGEVITY WITH STRENGTH TRAINING

Most of us will agree that the quality of our life is at least as important as its duration. It doesn't matter how many candles are on our birthday cake, but it doesn't matter how we look, feel and act throughout our lives.

The average life expectancy is around 76 to 77 years. It could be much higher, even more than 100 years, but until recently, the lack of knowledge has allowed people to gradually eliminate their bodies, allowing them to decompose with age like an old car or a building.

Modern medicine is organized to treat symptoms with medication. It cannot and does not educate people to correct their dietary and metabolic defects to be healthier, stay young and live more.

Now we know that it is possible to improve almost all aspects of our body: muscle and bone mass, metabolic improvement, healing time, organ function and recover youthful appearance, changing our metabolism and the chemistry of our body.

Aging comes mainly from an alteration in the body's metabolism, which are the chemical processes that control growth, energy production, and waste disposal. When we are young, our metabolism works at a high level, and the body can restore, rebuild and repair tissues and systems quickly and efficiently.

As we approach midlife, weakened glands cause our hormonal levels to change and the brain receives signals from a weakened and faltering biological system and enters a gradual mode of "shutting down." It is assumed that the time has come to begin the process of eliminating this organism from the natural landscape and changing the metabolism in a catabolic way of decomposition and we are on the right path.

Studies have shown that the most common factor in long-term people worldwide is maintaining their muscle mass. This suggests that your metabolism is more oriented towards growth and repair, as well as the fact that your lifestyle is active.

It is easy to replicate this situation with an appropriate training program that contains at least 60 percent of strength training exercises to keep muscles intact for life.

Instead of a degenerative, toxic and flaccid shell destined to be gradually eliminated, the correct exercise forces the rejuvenation of a healthy body by telling the brain to change the metabolism. The best hormonal secretions of healthy glands instruct the brain not to go into "off" mode or can prevent this from happening if it is already in progress.

Proper exercise as strength training releases the natural human growth hormone. This is a protein hormone that is very useful for rejuvenating the body, restoring energy levels and strengthening the immune system by reducing the risk of some potentially lethal diseases that can eliminate it prematurely.

It has been shown that strength training exercise is more effective in stimulating the release of this growth hormone than any other form of exercise. To receive maximum benefits, be sure to get the help of a gym instructor or a fitness professional to set up your exercise program correctly. It is important to do things correctly; otherwise, it is unlikely that you can train at the appropriate level of intensity to stimulate the body to produce this "physical fitness hormone."

You will be rewarded with so many benefits that will surprise you. You can restore healthy levels of body fat, younger-looking skin, become stronger and fitter and enjoy higher energy levels that will make you feel 20 years younger. Therefore, better health and longevity will be yours for many years.

CHAPTER FOUR

START TAKING CARE OF YOUR SKIN EARLY TO STAY BEAUTIFUL WITH AGE

Many people seek beauty advice in the media. Advice gotten from media are sometimes unhealthy and media view of the world does not represent reality at all. You must create your understanding of beauty. Read on to discover tips and suggestions to become the most beautiful version of yourself.

Dark mascara is a fantastic trick to use if you want your eyes to look bigger. Disposable mascara sticks can be used to separate and define the eyelashes and remove excess lumps and mascara.

To reproduce the color of your splendid hazelnuts or splendid green eyes, choose darker neutrals that create contrast with lighter eyes, shades that have a red base to highlight green or other complementary shades. Try pewter silver, lavender, light brown or dark purple.

Try coconut oil instead of spending a lot of money on expensive skin moisturizers. Switch to using virgin coconut oil because it can easily penetrate the skin providing soothing hydration while reducing the appearance of fine lines and wrinkles. This also helps treat certain skin conditions, such as eczema, psoriasis, and acne, due to the natural antibacterial and antifungal properties it possesses.

Make sure makeup pencils are sharp. You must also ensure they are clean and safe to use. To make a liner effective and perfect for use, place it in the freezer for ten minutes and then sharpen it.

The brightness should only be used sparingly. This will create a pleasant light effect. Use it on the cheeks, nose and puffs, then apply loose powder on the top.

Fruit juices contain numerous vitamins for the skin. The consumption of fresh fruits and vegetables provides valuable nutrients. Including the juice of these foods in your diet is a tasty way to make sure you get the nutrients you need! Replace artificially sweetened beverages with juice and your skin will thank you.

Try using a vegetable sponge to remove skin imperfections. It helps to exfoliate and softens the skin. Using a vegetable sponge and an exfoliating body scrub gives you twice the benefits. You should use vegetable sponge a few times a week.

Always remember that beauty is often subjective. If you have confidence, health and care for yourself, then you are already beautiful. Ignore those who hate you and never doubt that you are beautiful inside and out!

Be sure to shave and then exfoliate before applying any tanning spray. If you are concerned about preparing the skin in advance, the color will be applied more evenly and is more likely to appear natural.

Eye drops can add shine to your eyes during the day. This will reduce that tired look and make you look refreshed. Always keep it on your desk at work and follow the package instructions.

To reduce the appearance of swelling of the face from inside the mouth, place an ice cube in the mouth and hold it on the palette with your tongue. This will make your face swell less by relaxing it. Then splash your face with cold water and you will find that you have a remedy for that swollen appearance.

Some people's beauty regimes tend to establish themselves at a certain age as they get used to doing things familiarly and comfortably. There is nothing wrong with doing so as long as it makes you happy. However, if you plan to look for a job again or if you are wondering how it can look better, it is worth taking the time to consult a trusted beautician or friend. It is also worth considering changing your routine a bit. If you are becoming less happy with the results of your regular routine, you may consider seeking the help of an injectable expert.

Lotion is very important to moisturize all skin types. It is good for many things. Not only can the lotion repair dry skin immediately, it can also resolve an emergency of curly hair. Apply a small amount of lotion on your palms and smooth over your hair.

To get a good manicure, apply nail polish in this order: 1 / Base Coat 2 / A pair of hands of the color you prefer 3 / A top coat. Do it about two hours before retiring at night. It is fine if it is not very clean and comes in contact with the skin. In the morning, the nails will be completely dry and it will be easy to remove any enamel from the skin with a light wash and rub. With these simple methods, you can do your pedicure and manicure quite well.

Apply some egg on your face to make your skin more beautiful. There are numerous benefits obtained from the consumption of eggs. You can also use eggs to improve your external beauty. You must break some eggs in a small bowl, then spread the mixture on your face. After letting the egg dry on your face, which will take up to 20 minutes, rinse it with warm water. That will help remove the oil on your face.

EXERCISE, ANTI-AGING AND LONGEVITY

Virtually everyone knows that exercise is an important component of good health. Many people know that cardiovascular exercise can help prevent heart disease, but the benefits of exercise go much further.

CARDIO WORKOUT: In a study of 17,000 Harvard alumni for a period of 30 years, it was found that moderate exercise, such as jogging, swimming or playing tennis, reduced the overall death rate by 25-33%, and not just for illness but For all causes of death. It is interesting to note that intense physical exercise, such as marathons, increase the mortality rate due to damage to the body caused by oxidative stress.

POWERFUL TRAINING: Strength training can also help you stay young. Have you ever noticed that older people tend to have less muscle mass than young people? As people get older and less hormones related to muscle growth are secreted, less muscle protein is produced, which can lead to the loss of lean muscle mass. This trend is exacerbated by the modern lifestyle, which does not incorporate strength strengthening as a natural result of daily activities.

LOSS OF MUSCLE MASS: Once the muscle mass is lost, the metabolic syndrome begins. Muscle mass is one of the main determining factors to establish the body's metabolic rate. When the metabolic rate decreases, people tend to gain weight in the abdominal region, which increases insulin resistance and possibly diabetes. Therefore, to reduce or reverse the wastage of lean muscle mass and the problems associated with aging, strength training is necessary.

FLEXIBILITY TRAINING: And let's not forget to stretch. During strength training, it is important to stretch before and after and not simply prevent muscle injuries. Stretching allows blood and nutrition to flow to the muscles. It also helps eliminate waste products produced in the muscles during exercise, preventing pain. Finally, stretching increases the range of motion, which allows you to recruit more muscle fibers during strength training, resulting in a greater increase in exercise muscle mass.

HOW DOES ANTI-AGING LONGEVITY AFFECT SEX?

Aging is an insidious process that slowly affects the biological process. The fact that the changes happen so slowly does not change the fact that the changes really take place.

In the past, aging has involved many theories about how this natural phenomenon occurs in all human beings. Most aging theories are based on the wear we see in everyday life. The elderly, as well as mechanical devices, often seem worn.

Human aging has two basic types.

1) Chronological aging applies to the number of candles a person has had on their birthday cake.

2) Biological aging is the real change in your body as it ages chronologically.

No one can change their chronological age, but each individual will have a different level of biological aging.

The science of anti-aging longevity is the process that slows the biological aging process. Now we have found a way not only to delay aging, but in many cases, they have managed to reverse the effect of chronological aging.

THEORIES OF AGING

There are several theories about aging. One of the most common arguments accepted today is the fact that aging is inherent in its genes. As genetics and DNA are better understood, it becomes an important aspect of what one might expect from longevity. Of course, the better you take care of yourself, the more you get close to reaching your genetically programmed maximum.

Observations have proven that people in high-stress conditions age faster than those who are not so exposed. Stress has been shown to affect the hormonal production of the hypothalamus. Each time the production of hormones in the body is disturbed, the regeneration process will not work properly and will lead to premature aging.

The theory of wear on the problem of aging derives from the observation of mechanical devices that will eventually wear out. This theory does not put into consideration the body's ability to repair itself and the regeneration of living tissues.

The theory of free radicals is the most widely accepted explanation of aging. Free radicals or highly reactive body chemicals are the main cause of tissue damage. These free radicals have several uses in the body. However, many of these body chemicals can damage our cells and tissues. These chemicals are looking for additional electrons. This allows them to steal electrons from other molecules. As they continue to do so, they eventually damage our cells in our bodies and create new harmful chemicals in the process.

EFFECTS OF AGING ON SEX

We experience different changes as we age. These changes can be both psychological and physical. Our sexual vigor is undoubtedly one of the things that change when we age. During our youth, we have unlimited energy and enthusiasm for this activity. With age, we tend to lose the urge, drive and our ability to have sex starts to wane as we grow older.

The hormonal changes that are normal during the aging process can significantly affect the levels of our sexual desire. In men, testosterone decreases due to aging and any health condition. It is similar in women since many studies show that the desire of many women decreases with age.

How to maintain sexual desire

A more effective way to improve sexual desire with age is to have regular sex. Keeping your body fit and healthy, regular and satisfying sexual performance can really train your body to respond well to sex.

Learning the changing psychology of sex as you get older can also help you and your partner have a more satisfying sexual relationship. It is necessary to consider existing drugs, stable medical conditions, adequate preliminary and appropriate positions. Given these factors, you will surely have a more satisfying sexual experience.

Smart supplement

Taking a multivitamin can help you stay healthy. But two nutrients that are not usually found in your daily vitamin consumption can improve physical and mental health. The first is Rhodiola, a natural herb natively belonging to Siberia. Researchers are aware that Rhodiola is a wonderful adaptogen that can mitigate the repercussion of anxiety and stress. But now, other medical researchers have discovered that it can also improve physical and cognitive deficiencies in the elderly.

During their study, 120 adults, between 50 and 89 years of age with physical and cognitive deficits, received a multivitamin and Rhodiola supplement. A group of 62 patients took both capsules after eating breakfast. The other group took only one tablet after taking breakfast and another after lunch. Both groups experienced an impressive improvement in motivation, alertness, libido, sleep quality, concentration, memory and mood, the group that took the full dose of Rhodiola at breakfast found a greater impact. The usual recommendation is 200 to 600 mg. of Rhodiola per day. Look for a standardized extract of 0.78% rosavin.

L-carnitine is a supplement that can improve mental and physical health because it contributes to energy metabolism and improves the function of neurotransmitters in the brain. In a recent study, centenarians, who took 2,000 mg. L-carnitine for six months registered significant improvements in mental and physical fatigue and muscle mass. 250 mg intake every day or 550 mg. in a few days on a weekly basis works for most people. L-carnitine is particularly useful for vegetarians, as it is found only in small amounts in vegetables, fruits and legumes.

Increase your daily diet

When it comes to eating for longevity and wellbeing, you want the most nutritious foods on your plate. But as we get older, eating healthy becomes more stimulating. The caloric requirement decreases as nutritional requirements increases. What is the solution? Go for healthy foods that offer the most nutrients for the least amount of calories. The problem is that health experts have not yet agreed on what makes up a nutrient-rich food. Some stores and food manufacturers have developed their own nutritional guidance systems, creating confusion rather than clarification. To simplify diet and food intake, the FDA is considering a national system for classifying and labeling food. But it could be years before there is a unified system.

Meanwhile, here is a simple rule to buy: look for the least processed foods you can find. You will find many nutrient-rich foods in the store. Buy the aisles at the end and don't spend much time there.

Do you need something a little more directed? Here are some healthy and nutrient-rich foods to include to your longevity shopping list:

Fruits: apricots, bananas, berries, melon, grapes, kiwi, mango,

 oranges, papayas, peaches, pomegranates, and watermelons

Vegetables: broccoli, Brussels sprouts, carrots, cauliflower, green leafy vegetables such as black cabbage, romaine lettuce and spinach, peppers, sweet potatoes and tomatoes

Meat, chicken, fish, eggs: eggs, lean meat, pork loin, salmon and chicken without skin or turkey breast

Dairy products: cheese (lean), ricotta (lean), milk (lean or thin), yogurt (lean or thin)

Bread, cereals, cereals: amaranth, barley, 100% whole wheat bread, brown rice, bulgur, bran, oats and oats, 100% whole wheat pasta, quinoa, spelled tortillas and whole wheat

Canned foods: beans and lentils, fruits (in water or own juices), sardines, organic soup reduced in sodium, light tuna packed in water and tomatoes

Frozen foods: fruits, vegetables (without sauce), vegetarian burgers and whole waffles.

Packaged appetizers: nuts, unsalted nuts, sautéed popcorn, pumpkin seeds and sunflower seeds

Condiments and condiments: fruit creams, hummus, low-fat salad dressing and sauce

Oils and spices: flaxseed and flaxseed oil, organic herbs and spices, extra virgin olive oil, tomato sauce, walnut oil

Drinks: 100% fruit juice, low sodium vegetables or tomato juice

How to reduce the aging process with strength training exercise

Your body is the only possession that you fully possess. There may be some spare parts available today, but there are no substitutes. Land, houses, cars, money and other assets can be acquired, but they can be lost. You can take all these things away, but only death can steal your body.

The state of your body determines your lifestyle to a devastating degree. Without a healthy, strong, fit and vital body, all other goods become useless. You can ask yourself:

"If this is really the only body I will have, do I want it to work well?

"Do I really want to stay strong, active, young and healthy physically and mentally?"

"Do I want to maintain total mobility and, therefore, independence throughout my life?"

"I think it's something that I have something to say or something about which I can do something."

"Am I ready to invest some time and effort to stay as young as possible for as long as possible?"

Everyone seeks the magic answer and a quick solution, but most ignore the good science that already exists and is well proven. Each of us has the key to our fountain of youth that so many people are looking for; we just need to open the door and enter.

The secret is the right exercise. Physical strength and fitness are the key to health and longevity and is the closest thing to a "magic bullet" to ensure the absence of diseases, longevity, and high quality of life.

Many people in our so-called civilized nations pursue an accelerated aging program that makes them feel old and exhausted long before their time and increases the 50% risk of contracting a disease that could shorten their lives. This program is best characterized by waist expansion, muscle contraction, loss of strength and fitness, decreased thinking power, increased blood pressure, pain and aches, reduced energy and increased general feeling of fatigue.

If you want to accelerate the aging process and shorten your life, the way to do it is to do what most people are already doing: avoid exercise, eat a large percentage of your diet from food sold in beautiful boxes made with ingredients cheap ground that has no nutritional content, lie on the couch, watch TV, drink beer and eat french fries in your spare time and aging disabilities will reach you faster than you can imagine.

It does not always have to be so, a program that includes strength training exercises performed only twice a week can completely stop and even reverse this ticket to nothing.

Ask yourself the above questions and if the answers are yes, get stuck and start an appropriate training program. Request the help of a fitness professional at your local gym to set up your program and teach you the correct training technique. It is also imperative that you perform your exercises with the appropriate intensity level since, without them, you are unlikely to obtain significant results.

The world has constantly sought the fountain of youth for centuries. We want to survive but also want to look younger, feel younger, be active and live a fuller, richer and healthier life. Everything is waiting for you to grab it, then stretch and take it.

The power of enzymes: by digestion, absorption of nutrients and longevity

Overeating or eating the wrong foods can cause bodily reactions such as excess gas and acids, bloating and stiffness. Do you often need an antacid after eating certain types of food? If you know what I mean here, the problem is probably due to a diet based on highly processed or overcooked foods.

This type of food is not digestible, and your body simply cannot eliminate it efficiently. Indigestible food is the food to which all natural enzymes have been removed and other healthy nutrients removed. The lack of enzymes in food is also known as denatured food. Enzymes are what cause the ripening, deterioration and decay of the fruit. Have you ever noticed how margarine is not spoiled? There is no enzyme present; it is not digestible; it is not healthy for your body.

Enzymes are essential catalysts for healthy chemical reactions within the body. In other words, enzymes are protein-based substances that bind to other nutrients that cause changes in the body by accelerating activities such as food digestion, nutrient absorption, and tissue maintenance and repair. More than 2000 different enzymes play an active role in digestion and many other essential body functions.

Enzymes work effectively in perfect harmony with other necessary nutrients called cofactors such as vitamins, minerals, essential fatty acids and phytochemicals.

The perfect natural complex requires the presence of all other players in the team or the game is not taking place. This could be the main reason why supplementation with synthetic and non-integral vitamins with dietary vitamins or supplementation with other nutrients alone does not work. No nutrient without the others will be the only magic bullet. Nature is more complex than that. Therefore, enzymes without cofactors will have no activity.

The average modern diet is made up of foods that are too elaborate, lack nutrients and overcook. Warming any whole food above 118 degrees F destroys enzymes and other important healthy nutrients. A good rule to follow to get more enzymes is; raw before cooking, steamed vegetables before boiling, drowned before boiling and cooking rare meats before cooking them well.

Experts believe that 82 percent of our energy consumed goes to digest a typical cooked and processed meal. Our overloaded digestive system works 24 hours a day, 7 days a week, trying to break down foods that, for the most part, are not digestible or only partially digested. This could take days to get rid of a meal, or never!

Due to this continuous process, only about 20 percent of the body's energy remains to handle other vital functions such as thinking, breathing, vision and immune system support, just to name a few. It's like this if you want to stay healthy or be healthier, you need to get more out of your digestive and elimination process.

Regardless of the amount of trans fat, the amount of white sugar and flour or any other non-digestible substance that you can ingest, your body will try to break it down with enzymes. Foods that are easy to digest and eliminate in the body are raw or natural whole food. Your body will not have to use so much energy to produce enough digestive enzyme juices to convert food into a usable halfway.

Most modern societies consume food that was never intended to produce a healthy body. We know that over the centuries, we have not evolved as a species when eating foods such as hamburgers, french fries, pizza, soda and beer. Our digestive system simply cannot break down these chemical pumps. This material is not completely digested and, without enzymatic activity, will remain in the intestine forever, rotting.

Over time, part of these leaks out of the intestine and escapes into the bloodstream by taxing the entire body. The organs of the body that have never been thought to eliminate toxins try to do exactly that. Organs like the kidneys, lungs and skin can become inflamed and sick in an attempt to eliminate toxic waste from a poor diet and an inadequate digestive process — the unfortunate consequences of overcooked fast food and whole food diets.

Choosing to eat healthier involves eating more food in its raw form or eating lightly cooked food. Eating one meal a day with this knowledge in mind helps your body in a more productive process of elimination and digestion.

Ideally, we should eat 80 percent of our food this way, but unfortunately, this probably won't happen to most people. What can you do to support this important process in your body and get rid of a large amount of accumulated sludge in the intestinal tract?

By integrating with a good digestive enzyme supplement product found at any local health food store, you will make a wise decision to improve your overall health.

Each of us can benefit from this special knowledge, from the elderly to young children. We must return what is not in our food. This is much cheaper than going to your local doctor, who has never studied much about the enzymes at the medical school. Some doctors treat diseases by masking the symptoms with medications.

Enzyme supplements are a simple solution for a wide range of health problems. If you had a doctor who told you that your diet is physically damaging you and that you are sacrificing your longevity through the food you are eating daily, then it would not make sense if the same doctor that you use food and drink to restore your physical condition. However, if you know exactly how your diet has damaged your health, then you will know how to use it to correct the anomaly. My advice is you should not always rely on doctors to know how, since they have been trained to use drugs, surgery and other intrusive measures.

IS AN ANTI-AGING DIET GOOD FOR YOU?

No matter if you want to hear it or not, a balanced diet against aging is one of the best tools for your skin and health benefits against aging. The basis is simple. If you give your body the nutrients and adequate fuel it needs, you will get optimal results.

There are many anti-aging foods, anti-aging supplements, anti-aging vitamins that will help you ensure a well-balanced diet in your fight against the aging process.

Consider your car, for example. If you do not supply it with the right type of fuel, it will consume faster. It will not work as well, you will not get the correct fuel efficiency and it will probably not last long. If you give it the best possible fuel, on the other hand, you will see that it works longer, better and has fewer problems.The same thing works for your body. Your body needs all the right nutrients if you want to do what you want it to do and provide the right level of anti-aging possibilities. Many people make the mistake of looking for another way to improve their condition instead of looking at their individual needs.

Instead of striving to improve health through practical means, such as a healthy diet against aging, they look for other solutions that could be easier to achieve. However, there is simply nothing more effective than controlling what you eat for the health of your body.

WHAT YOUR BODY REQUIRES

For your body to have a healthy diet against aging, it requires a high level of nutrients and a low level of saturated fats and sugars. For example, you need vegetables. Most vegetables contain high levels of nutrients and also provide the right amount of antioxidants, which help stimulate cells, improve blood circulation and eliminate toxins from the body.

This, in itself, is an element that needs to improve its aging. A perfect way to get more of these in your diet is by squeezing vegetables. Replace your drinks with vegetable drinks (prepare them yourself to add nutrients and reduce costs.)

You should also eliminate anything that can cause potential problems from your diet. For example, sugars can cause health complications because they produce insulin. Insulin is an accelerator of aging and something you don't need in your diet. By minimizing the amount of sugar you eat, you inadvertently reduce the amount of insulin, which reduces the effects of aging on your body. There are now many specific anti-aging foods that will help you improve your diet.

Taking a look at how you can improve your diet, you can get some of the best anti-aging solutions for your health.

ANTI-AGING DIET: THE DEFINITIVE APPROACH

The last anti-aging diet should include foods as natural as possible, both in form and in consumption. Fried foods, sugars, heavily processed foods should be eliminated. They are part of an "aging diet" because they lead directly to make it look and age, not to mention the fact that they are the cause of many ailments and diseases that people face.

The reality is that the only form of diet that will promote the prevention of looking and feeling older, and that in reality will have the ability to reverse many elements that the aging process has already implemented. Many anti-aging diet composed of so many natural-based foods, especially in fruits and vegetables. This anti-aging diet should also be consumed raw to provide these extremely beneficial results.

At first it can be difficult to swallow the idea that – to reverse the aging process, to look and feel much younger – you will have to follow an anti-aging diet that is essentially a raw vegan diet. At first, it may seem extreme, but you will soon realize that the benefits of eating raw are not only obvious enough, but they are vital for staying healthy, staying healthy and freeing yourself from the disease.

The good thing about it is that many people follow this type of anti-aging diet and benefit from it. Once you've explored the raw vegan landscape, you'll soon discover the incredible selection of foods and recipes available.

There are also incredible desserts that taste a thousand times better than any traditional dessert filled with processed sugar. And the basic foods of an anti-aging diet based on raw vegetables are really very tasty and abundant.

Beyond the typical world of processed food wastes, sugar-rich foods, there is a world in which natural foods are kings and create powerful, healthy, vibrant and disease-free individuals. It is really the anti-aging diet par excellence and the anti-aging lifestyle to follow.

Are you ready for an anti-aging diet?

The anti-aging diet can slow down the harmful effects of aging caused by free radicals. People who follow a diet rich in antioxidants have aged relatively slower than those who do not. Fruits and especially green vegetables are rich in antioxidants. They help the body to neutralize free radicals and delay the aging procedure.

The ability of the body to manufacture digestive enzymes reduces as it ages. We must include in our diet the foods that will help in the production of digestive enzymes such as vitamin C and alpha-lipoic acid. Green tea and coffee varieties are rich in antioxidants. Cranberries, blueberries and artichokes are just some of the fruits and vegetables that are high in antioxidants.

At a certain age, a diet sufficient in refined sugar and wheat can cause hyperglycemia which is attributed to skin aging in some people. The type of sugar present in refined sugar and wheat can cause the skin to lose elasticity and, therefore, cause the skin to sag and wrinkle.

An anti-aging diet is a diet rich in antioxidants that make the body younger. An anti-aging diet should not include fats, especially unsaturated ones and must have more vegetables. Fats should be eliminated from the average diet.

The unsaturated fats of these foods are such an important factor that influences the aging process. In addition, these are the same foods to which we attribute the loss of energy, diseases and even fatal diseases.

These foods are generally of the fried and fatty type, such as junk food and the fast and fatty food diet. On the contrary, keep healthy fats such as olive oils and fish.

Antioxidant foods prevent heart disease and the development of most cancers, in addition to curbing the effects of aging. Some of the antioxidant foods that should be included in an anti-aging diet are blueberry berries, raspberries, blackberries and goji berries. It has been discovered that tomatoes have a high content of omega 3, which is a strong antioxidant substance.

Broccoli, spinach and carrots are some of the richest antioxidant vegetables. Eating them raw prevents the loss of nutrients inherent in cooking. Eating raw vegetables is an excellent anti-aging diet.

How an anti-aging diet can make you look younger

Everyone wants to find the secret ingredient to reverse aging and make people look younger. Unfortunately, contrary to what these anti-aging fashions come and go regularly, it is simply not possible for a single ingredient to reverse all the effects of aging. The reality is that aging is not caused by just one thing. It is caused by a complex range of problems that affect everyone in different ways and to varying degrees.

That is why the only way to fight against the effects of aging is to adopt a multifaceted approach. Instead of taking a magic pill or buying an overrated exercise device, you should turn it into a way of life. In short, in addition to daily exercise, you must follow an anti-aging diet.

Antioxidants: The most critical part of an anti-aging diet is eating foods that keep your body's cells functioning at youth levels. One of the ways to do it is to consume many antioxidants. If there is a magic ingredient in the anti-aging diet, these are the only ones. In non-technical terms, antioxidants fight free radicals, which are small molecules that bounce inside cells, causing all kinds of damage. Antioxidants eliminate these annoying things, allowing cells to function cleanly and renew without interference.

Different foods are excellent sources of antioxidants, some of which are blueberries, blueberries, tomatoes, grapes, garlic, carrots, whole grains, dark chocolate, green tea and red wine. Some daily portions of one of these foods are an essential part of an anti-aging diet.

Fatty acids: Omega-3 fatty acids help keep the body running smoothly in different ways, which makes them another important ingredient in an anti-aging diet. First, they act as a lubricant, not very different from the oil in the car, helping the joints move and blood flow easily. They also help maintain healthy cells by strengthening cell walls and increasing the functioning of the cognitive and nervous system by providing a fluid medium for the passage of nerve signals.

If you want healthy fatty acids to be a component of your anti-aging diet, eat a lot of fish, especially salmon, anchovies, mackerel, sardines, herring, flax seeds, chia seeds, soybeans, egg whites, and vegetable oils.

Other important ingredients in an anti-aging diet

Fruits and vegetables, in addition to their ability to provide many antioxidants, also contain many vitamins and fiber.

Whole grains provide abundant dietary fiber, which helps reduce blood cholesterol levels and also contain healthy doses of protein and other nutrients.

Legumes have low calories while they contain many proteins, particularly when mixed with complementary ingredients such as corn and whole grains.

Yogurt is excellent for eliminating bacteria and other toxins that accumulate in the bloodstream and digestive tract, which will help your body run smoothly.

Nuts, in addition to containing many vitamins that help the brain develop, also provide a large amount of elastin and collagen, which help reduce wrinkles.

Information on anti-aging diets

You do not need to discard thousands of green tickets to stay young or age gracefully. In fact, surgery can only delay so much. If you do not focus on your diet and general health, you will grow old and may even develop some serious medical problems. After all, gravity is still gravity and life is still life: it will end at some point. If you are interested, an anti-aging diet can add years to your life and make you feel much younger than you. You do not have to keep yourself hungry or chew the bark to keep cool. Instead, if you focus on health, eat balanced meals and know what to put in your mouth, you could be as fit as you used to be. Here are some dietary anti-aging tips that can make you feel as good as you look.

Water and antioxidants: If the skin dries, wrinkles will appear. If your body is lacking water and the necessary nutrients, it will not work properly. Therefore, you should always endeavor to have enough water daily. You should take at least 5 or 6 cups of water a day to keep your skin hydrated and the circulation up and up. The key to any anti-aging diet is to make sure your body works in the best way. Water can guarantee it.

Antioxidants are a vital element of any anti-aging diet because they release poisons from the body and protect the immune mechanism of an individual. And, of course, natural antioxidants keep the body stable and skin shiny. Therefore, you should do everything possible to consume at least five servings a day of fruits and vegetables, such as onions, shallots and spinach, and you should do everything possible to consume tea. If you consume a cup or 2 of green tea a day, you can listen and see the results in no time! If you want to look young, you should consume whole grains and fish.

Whole grains and fish: These items will be part of any anti-aging diet sanctioned by the doctor. Fish is not only full of useful nutrients such as trans-omega-3 acids, but it is also an anti-inflammatory. Therefore, you won't have to worry about things like swollen ankles or a swollen-looking face.

Whole grains are a great piece of any anti-aging diet because they provide people with the fibers they need to keep their digestive tract in good condition. Therefore, you can be sure to digest food properly. Furthermore, this part of an anti-aging diet will keep cholesterol levels low, improving overall health.

ANTI AGING DIET - SECRETS

An anti-aging diet plan does not necessarily mean eating only raw foods or having to give up everything you love. It merely means selecting which foods are best for you. You can still choose from a long list of foods that will actively support your body and help you in your quest to look younger. Wouldn't it be great if you had the knowledge and experience that happened over the years, but you could leave wrinkles and diseases? If you are careful with your food, that dream may be closer than you think.

You can start your anti-aging food strategy just to understand which foods are healthy and which ones can age. Let's take a closer look at these things at this time.

Most green vegetables contain many antioxidants. Oxidants accelerate the aging process; Antioxidants defend themselves against them, that's why we want many antioxidants. Generally, it is safe to have several raw vegetables and salads whenever they are washed or peeled properly. Some of your vitamins and minerals may be lost during cooking. Fresh fruit is also rich in vitamins and minerals; therefore, include these foods in your diet as much as possible.

Lean proteins will develop muscles, which we tend to suffer as we age. Therefore, you will want low-fat portions of poultry, fish, pork, etc. in your anti-aging diet plan. Meat has many unwanted fats and, therefore, may not be a good option when someone ages. Most types of cheese are also high in saturated fats, so vegetarians should plan to get most of the protein from beans, with small portions of nuts and seeds.

You might also consider adding a supplement to your anti-aging diet program. Vitamins are necessary for the body to repair and renew itself, making you look younger. Calcium can strengthen bones and things like folic acid also help with mental alertness. Try to look for a supplement designed specifically for an anti-aging diet program or for people of a certain age.

Stay away from sugar if you can. A large amount of sugar can cause fluctuations in blood sugar levels which the body will find difficult to moderate as we age. This can be a cause of dangerous medical conditions like diabetes and it certainly does not make us look younger. Try to reduce sugar consumption in your anti-aging diet program.

CHAPTER FIVE

THE BEST 4-WEEK ANTI-AGING DIET PROGRAM

A health plan for longevity or a life-prolonging diet can include different practices:

1. Nutrition and environmental detoxification.

2. Integration of vitamins and quality nutrients.

3. Herbal therapy

4. traditional Chinese medicine

5. Chiropractic care

6. Acupuncture

7. Aesthetic and rehabilitative therapeutic massage.

However, if you really desire to achieve longevity in your daily life, a healthy diet is essential. Therefore, nutrition, vitamins and quality nutritional supplements and other skincare products along with a happy lifestyle and exercise are essential.

The diet plan for longevity: A longevity diet plan is really more than a collection of practical nutritional guidelines. Follow the four simple guidelines listed below each week to review the existing diet and start eating healthy without all the drama of a typical weight loss diet, since a longevity diet itself is about maintaining the right amount of healthy calories.

WEEK 1 - DUPLICATE VEGETABLES - REDUCE MILK AND CHEESE

In the first week, you will drastically reduce dairy products such as cheese, milk and ice cream and focus on doubling vegetables while. Here is why:

Vegetables provide us with vitamins and antioxidants that protect our body from damage and the effects of aging. First, research has shown that supplements cannot be replaced with food in its full form for the same benefits.

Vegetables such as carrots or cauliflower are also excellent for filling with nutritious foods and having fewer calories. So avoid choking them with cheese or cream sauce!

Dairy products are good for babies and children who need foods high in calories and fat; For adults, it is football that we only need. Vegetables will kick you.

As we all know, dairy products add calories, increase cholesterol and even increase the risk of certain types of cancer. Therefore, eliminating dairy products from the diet will reduce the overall risk of these diseases.

Focus your attention on the first week. Buy and eat your favorite vegetables and you will not miss the dairy.

 The best vegetables:

 # Spinach

 # Lettuce

 # Peppers

 # Broccoli

Prepare them in olive oil with salt, pepper and other spices.

Remember no cheese in vegetables!

WEEK 2 - DEGRADE MEAT AND NUTS

Like dairy products, meat is not so good for you. Meat provides protein to your body, but not much else. Meat contains saturated fats (bad fats).

Nuts, on the other hand, contain good proteins and fats, including essential omega-3 fatty acids that regulate cholesterol and increase brain function in terms of mental clarity.

Vegetarians indeed have healthier arteries than those who eat meat. The second week focuses on reducing a source of protein (meat) and replacing it with another (nuts).

Continue to double your consumption of vegetables and eliminate dairy products while:

1. Decrease meat intake: think of meat as a side dish for sautéed vegetables. Do not use more than half the amount of meat you usually eat and opt for lean meats such as chicken and pork.

2. Nuts: rich in protein and healthy fats, nuts, almonds and nuts are excellent, providing your body with excellent nutrients, without salt and in its purest form.

QUICK ADVICE: put the nuts everywhere! Bring some bags of nuts in the car, at the desk, at home. Eat something when you're hungry, a handful per session is a good amount.

WEEK 3 - GET FISH, NOT WHITE FOOD

Add the fish to your diet and eliminate "white foods" such as white flour and refined sugar that are highly processed and contain almost no nutrients. Avoid non-whole grain products and avoid anything with added sugar.

Fish is good, contains omega-3, is rich in protein and essential fatty acids, lowers cholesterol and increases mental clarity.

Eat fish up to thrice weekly. Fish serves as an excellent meat substitute and is easy to prepare.

NOTE: some fish contain mercury and pesticides, so buy them locally if possible in a market, not in supermarkets where pesticides are used to prolong their shelf life and also contain saturated fats.

Some of the healthiest fish for longevity are considered salmon, sardines and anchovies.

WEEK 4 - LOVE FRUIT, AVOID CHEMICALS

The last week includes increasing the amount of fruit you eat while avoiding foods that may contain harmful chemicals.

The plan eats dessert fruit at least twice a day. This provides you with important antioxidants and vitamins, and be sure to wash the fruit, as it will contain pesticides and chemicals that could be harmful to your health and aid aging.

1. Enjoy the fruit: strawberries, blueberries and the resveratrol present in grapes can satisfy that sweet desire after dinner. Eat real fruit instead of fruit juices while increasing your blood sugar level. Avoid milkshakes made up of tons of calories. Eat a whole variety of fruit, the more colors, the better.

2. Avoid chemicals: "concentrated sugar" ingredients, such as high-fructose corn syrup, can directly cause an immediate metabolic syndrome and cause huge spikes in the risk of diabetes.

CHAPTER SIX

HEALTHY LIFESTYLE AND LONGEVITY

What exactly is a healthy lifestyle?

These five areas have been chosen because previous studies have shown influence premature death. This is how these healthy habits were defined and measured:

A healthy diet, which has been calculated and classified based on the informed intake of healthy foods such as vegetables, fruits, nuts, whole grains, healthy fats and omega-3 fatty acids and unhealthy foods such as red and processed meats, sugar Beverages, trans fats and sodium.

Level of healthy physical activity, measured daily with at least 30 minutes a day of moderate to vigorous activity.

Sound body weight is defined as a normal body mass index (BMI) between 18.4 and 24.

Moderate alcohol consumption, measured between 5 and 15 grams per day for women and 5 to 30 grams per day for men is advised. In general, a drink contains approximately 14 grams of pure alcohol. It is 12 ounces of regular beer, 5 ounces of wine or 1.5 ounces of spirits.

The researchers also analyzed data on age, ethnicity and drug use, as well as comparative data from national surveys on health and nutrition exams and large-scale online data from the Centers for Control and Prevention Diseases for epidemiological research.

Does a healthy lifestyle make a difference?

Healthy habits make a difference in human life. According to this analysis, people who met the criteria for the five habits enjoyed significantly longer lives than those who had none: 14 years for women and 12 years for men (if they had these habits at the age of 50). People who did not have any of these habits were much more likely to die prematurely from cancer or cardiovascular disease.

The study researchers also calculated life expectancy based on how many of these five healthy habits people had. Only a healthy habit (and no matter which one) only one prolonged the life expectancy of two years in men and women. As expected, the healthier habits they have had, the longer they last.

A study in 2018 showed that people over 50 years who had a normal weight, had never smoked and drunk alcohol in moderation, lived on average seven more years. A 2012 mega analysis of 15 international studies involving more than 500,000 participants found that more than half of premature deaths were due to unhealthy lifestyle factors such as poor diet, inactivity, obesity, excessive alcohol consumption and smoking And the list of ongoing research support.

KEY THINGS YOU CAN DO TO LIVE MORE AND ENJOY A LONGER LIFE SPAN

It is disappointing that we cannot drink from the fabulous fountain of youth, but the good news is that most of us are born with a good dose of long life: only about 25% of age-related diseases are genetically determined. This means that our environment and our lifestyle choices are much stronger predictors of how long we will live. In most cases, these are factors that we can significantly influence. Small changes in lifestyle may not seem extraordinary, but they have a great advantage. Consider the potential of physical exercise to increase your longevity: the heart and lungs of a couch potatoes' heart and lungs carry about 2 percent less oxygen in the rest of the body a year after age 30, while a person of the same age who burns 3000 calories per week through aerobic exercise can expect to lose only half of one percent of their heart and lung capacity each year (at least until the age of 80 or 90 years). Since every single cell in our body needs oxygen to function and stay healthy, this unique lifestyle difference resolves a possible -year difference in longevity.

Most of the decisions and actions we need to live a long and healthy life is common sense, and in part it is fun. Although some suggestions may seem simple, their impact can be enormous.

People who exercise regularly live between 5 and 7 years longer than those who are inactive. Exercise, such as walking, strengthens your bones. Aerobic exercise strengthens your heart. Write down at least 30 minutes of activity on most days.

EVALUATE YOUR WEIGHT: Obesity, which is related to heart disease, type 2 diabetes and other health conditions, reduces life expectancy, but the increased risk of dying prematurely is not limited only to those who are technically obese (defined by an index of body mass or BMI, 30 or more). Most people with a BMI greater than 25 also have a higher mortality rate than people whose weight is in a healthy range. (Experts speculate that they may also engage in unhealthy behaviors, such as smoking and overeating, more frequently.) Talk to your doctor about what is healthy for you: ranges vary by sex and height.

DO NOT SMOKE: People who smoke during adulthood, expose themselves to tons of harmful and dangerous chemicals and end up dying about nine years earlier than they would have naturally died. The good thing about it is that quitting smoking can add most of those years.

SLEEP INSUFFICIENCY: Sleeping well at night can help reduce stress, keep weight in a healthy range and give you energy for the next day. Record at least seven hours per night. When you get enough sleep, your body repairs and regenerates weak and/or dead tissues, and strengthens your immune system as well.

MAKE POOLS: Taking a nap for 30 minutes a day could reduce the risk of heart disease by up to 30 percent, according to research from the Harvard School of Public Health. Scientists suspect that a daily nap lowers stress hormones in the body. (Just don't rely on these regularly to compensate for not having enough clock hours during the night).

TAKE ATTENTION IF YOU DRINK ALCOHOL: While some studies have proven that moderate alcohol consumption (one drink per day or less for women, two drinks per day or less for men) can contribute to longevity in some people, beer, wine and spirits. They certainly have their negative side. In addition to the health risks associated with excessive alcohol consumption, it is among the top five sources of calories for American adults, which contributes to weight gain. If you are one who enjoys a good glass of wine, make sure you do it in moderation.

EAT WELL: Enjoying a diet rich in fruits and vegetables, whole grains, low-fat dairy products and seafood is related to longevity. These foods provide heart-healthy vitamins, minerals, and fats that increase longevity and help fight against diseases.

MANAGING STRESS: Chronic stress creates an avenue for many health conditions. Stress probably exerts its adverse effects by triggering an inflammatory reaction of our immune system. Meditation, massage and gentle forms of exercise, such as yoga, for example, can help reduce stress.

GET VITAMIN D: People who have higher levels of vitamin D can live up to five more years, according to a study by researchers at King's College London; They concluded that the part of our chromosomes that shortens with age might not be reduced as quickly as it would if the levels were lower. The best source of vitamin D is a good old-fashioned sun, so try to spend 15 minutes outdoors almost every day.   Shiitake mushrooms, fortified cereals and fatty fish such as salmon and tuna are some good food sources of vitamin D, but getting it from a variety of places is essential, says Mark Liponis, MD, a doctor at Canyon Ranch (1994-2018). Talk to your specialist about a vitamin D supplement if you think you are low.

TRANSFORM THE INTIMATE A PRIORITY: Studies suggest that having sex more frequently could prolong your life. Researchers at the West University of Scotland in Paisley have found that couples who have committed to having more sex for two weeks have registered lower blood pressure levels during stressful situations, such as public speaking, than couples who do. They refrain from having sex or have touched but have not had sex with him.   Low blood pressure levels indicate that your heart is not working hard to pump blood throughout the body, which helps prevent heart disease.

HOLD YOUR HANDS, EYE AND HUG: Even pampering counts. In a research study, researchers at Brigham Young University in Salt Lake City formed 18 couples to improve their partner's mood awareness by touching their necks, shoulders and hands reflexively, but not sexually. Another 18 couples received no guidance. Within a week, couples trained with a warm touch had higher levels of oxytocin, a wellness hormone; In addition, the men of these couples recorded lower levels of amylase, an indicator of stress. Lowering stress levels can help reduce the risk of a variety of health conditions.

PLACE THE SEAT BELT: Seat belts save lives: in 2010 alone, more than 12,000 people survived traffic accidents because they wore seat belts.

FLOSS YOUR TEETH REGULARLY: Flossing every night can eliminate bacteria that might otherwise cause gum inflammation. This inflammation activates the body's inflammatory response, which increases blood pressure (among other things) and increases the risk of having heart disease. That can potentially cause damage to the brain tissue, increasing the risk of developing diseases.

STAY CONNECTED: People with strong social networks (family, friends, clubs and groups) live longer lives than those who are not connected with others. The researchers hypothesize that the unhealthy impact of the stress hormone cortisol is reduced when people have friends and family to rely on.

DO NOT SKIP THE CHECKS: Regular checks can help identify potential problems early. The sooner a condition such as diabetes or hypertension is diagnosed and treated, the healthier it will be.

THE IMPORTANCE OF GOOD POSTURE IN AGING

Virtually every part of the body deteriorates at some point. It is all part of the aging process that is inevitable for everyone, regardless of their height in life. Carrying or lifting things now becomes a conscious effort; even simple things like climbing stairs or sitting can be daunting.

What occurs in our bodies as we age?

When you reach 50 or 60, you will probably notice something strange. You may notice a difference of half an inch or an inch in your height. This is a natural process caused by the narrowing of the spine.

The column is composed of vertebrae and among them, some discs act as a cushion. Over time, these discs lose their shape and begin to lose weight. Add to this, cartilage and connective tissues lose thickness and elasticity. All these things may not be aesthetically obvious at first. However, this could have been avoided if we take good care of our body through proper posture, healthy eating and regular exercise.

Posture is something that not everyone takes seriously, but it is very important as it promotes an independent lifestyle and movement. Having a correct posture improves balance and symmetry. You can avoid having hunched shoulders, back pain and narrowing of the spine. In part, it also makes you look good and feel good. In general, having a good posture is a good indicator of the age that will age in your life.

What are the benefits of good posture for the elderly?

There are many health problems caused by poor posture and correcting the habit can do a lot. However, if you want to have a good posture, you have to start somewhere. The perfect place for good posture to start is the spine. Few people know that our column carries about 10 kg of weight every day. Once you lean forward, gravity pushes you even more by squeezing your spine. Follow a series of consequences.

On the one hand, this may be the cause of the headache. As you lean forward when sitting, the tension in the cervical vertebrae builds up, causing misalignment. And over time, misalignment causes blood vessels to pinch, which limits their ability to supply blood to the brain, which then promotes headaches and migraines.

Bad posture can cause back pain. While bending down, the muscles and ligaments of the back fight and are under pressure to maintain balance. Pulling the muscles, especially in the lumbar area where most of the weight is transported, causes back pain. Over time, this habit can cause rapid degeneration of the spine, which can lead to severe complications such as osteoarthritis, scoliosis and osteoporosis.

Bad posture also compresses internal organs, decreasing their functionality and efficiency. Studies also show that abandonment has an important effect on digestion and blood flow. For this reason, the elderly can develop high blood pressure or low metabolic rate and put them at risk of heart attack, stroke and even diabetes and obesity. In addition to this, the curvature of the back causes the rib cage to contract, allowing the lungs and heart to have limited space to function. Also, too much pressure exerted on the spine can press on important blood vessels, limiting the correct blood flow, which is essential to nourish and originate these vital organs.

Now that we know how our bad postural habits can cause enormous health risks for our body making a conscious effort to change this through postural training can change things. Proper posture can make the elderly not to experience chest pain, back pain, headaches yet make them experience better digestion. And if you're still not convinced, the additional benefits of good posture influence the mental state of an older person. It has been proven that sitting down or standing can promote positivity, which gives more confidence to our thoughts and to our decision-making process.

In one experiment, having a good posture showed that the elderly developed a better memory remembrance. Although this is not yet proof that the correct posture can delay the Alzheimer's process, having the spine properly aligned while standing or sitting makes neurotransmitters can communicate faster from the brain to each part of the body, facilitating retention of the memory.

Good posture can also eliminate depression. Sitting and walking in a straight line, energy levels have increased. People with poor posture are prone to panic, anxiety and shallow breathing, which makes it difficult to overcome negativity. A good posture improves circulation, oxygenates the body well and improves perception and positive thinking, leaving one still at peace and ready to face any problem that may arise from the path of the elderly. Participating in an exercise program for the elderly is a good way to start.

In fact, for older people, starting to think about their early posture can help them move forward in the aging process. And if the correct posture is complemented by regular exercise and a healthy diet, aging for any older person will be just another phase from which they can enjoy more and benefit.

FIVE YOGA POSITIONS THAT WILL REWARD YOU WITH LONGEVITY AND YOUNGER BODY

The human body is like a sacred temple where the soul resides. And what is true if the soul's home is not in good shape, fit and healthy? Unhappiness, complexity, laziness and diseases slowly begin to manifest and destroy what was once pure, fresh and stimulating.

Yoga, the ancient science of life that emanates from the Himalayan region has long been a "buzzword" when it comes to maintaining a healthy body. The holistic practice of yoga that encourages a natural way of life is actually a way of life rather than a simple discipline. Those who have the will and dedication to accept this harmonious lifestyle will have a healthy body, a calm mind and a pure soul.

The best: Yoga can be practiced by everyone, regardless of their age, religion, caste, color and race. Yoga unifies everything and teaches a person to live healthy, happy and spread love to others.

Now let's take a look at five yoga positions that will not only introduce a life of health and happiness but will also keep you young and energetic well beyond your advanced years.

Plow Pose (Halasana)

1. With your arms along the side of the body, lie on your back and the palms of your hands should face up.

2. Breathe deeply, lift your legs so that they are at right angles to your body.

3. Now hold your hips with your hands and remove them from the floor.

4. Place the feet behind the head and place them gently on top.

5. Your back should be perpendicular.

6. Hold for a minute and exhale slowly.

Halasana is one of the best yoga positions for anxiety and offers a lot of benefits that include better metabolism, weight loss, better digestion, less stress, more flexibility and more.

Warrior II (Virabhadrasana 2)

1. Stand straight with a few feet between your feet.

2. Turn the left foot inward and the right foot outward 90 degrees.

3. Raise your arms so they are on the same level as your shoulders. The palms of the hands should be up.

4. Inhale and exhale bending the right knee.

5. Look to the right by gently turning your head.

6. Gently push the pelvis down and stretch your arms.

7. Continue breathing and stay in bed for at least one minute.

8. Breathe while you leave the pose and let the air out while you drop your arms.

9. Repeat the same with the left leg.

In addition to stretching and strengthening the ankles and legs, the pose helps to stretch the groin, shoulders, lungs and chest. Increase endurance and help with infertility, osteoporosis, flat feet, sciatica and more.

Shoulder support (Salamba Sarvangasana)

1. Lie on your back with your arms at your sides and your legs straight. In one movement, lift the legs, back and buttocks so that the lower part of the body is supported by the elbows while the shoulders support the weight of the body.

2. Keep your elbows close to each other and keep your spine and legs straight.

3. Breathe deeply and stay in position for at least one minute.

4. Lower your knees and gently release the posture.

Shoulder support is a popular posture that helps calm the brain, relieve stress, stretch the shoulders and neck, tone the legs and buttocks, stimulate the prostate glands and more.

Tree Pose (Vrksasana)

i. Stand straight with your both arms resting on your side. Keep your left leg straight while you place your right foot inside your left thigh slowly. Take a deep breath, raise both arms above your head and join them in the "Namaste" position.

ii. Your eyes should be straight and the spine erect. Keep breathing and stay in position for a minute. Release and repeat gently on the other leg.

Tree Pose or Vrksasana improves balance, balance and posture. Asana also helps with neuromuscular coordination, loosens the hip joints, improves concentration and strengthens the eyes, shoulders and inner ears.

Chair positioning (Utkatasana)

i. With your feet placed a few meters away, get on the carpet. Tilt your arms forward with your palms facing down. The arms should be straight.

ii. Bend your knees gently. Imagine you are sitting in a chair. Take a comfortable position, keep the spine stretched and smile.

iii. Hold the position for a while and relax slowly. The asana is perfect for stretching the chest, spine and hips. In addition to toning the legs, Vrksasana helps with back pain and also stimulates the heart and diaphragm.

Practice yoga regularly and you will witness a great change in your health, mind and lifestyle.

CHAPTER SEVEN

YOGA: A SECRET TO LONGEVITY?

Many people associate yoga with the elderly, typically 3000-year-old Indian yogis or Western and sticky Westerners who try to stay fit or "burn that belly fat."

Many people who practice yoga are old. However, the truth is that people of all ages can participate in yoga or yoga-like activities to promote longevity and live well enough to be ridiculed as "3,000-year-old yogis."

Yoga has a long history of relationships with, and essentially IS, human beings who seek to find harmony and balance within themselves and with the world around them to lead a peaceful and full life. What does longevity mean? In a more philosophical but true sense, it is really the same; As people get older, we begin to worry more and more about things like peace, harmony and balance. When applied to aspects of our life such as diet and exercise, these things are exactly what gives us longevity.

Regardless of your personal history, skill level or strength or even how many arts you have, yoga can be used to keep your body fresh, young, flexible and healthy for years to come. It is literally for everyone and this is the main reason why it has become so accessible, especially in recent decades. However, being so adaptable and vast also facilitates the customization of yoga for you and your body, which helps keep all kinds of people healthy and active.

But why does yoga promote longevity so well? What helps us so much?

Power: First, yoga helps us build strength throughout the body. One of the main reasons why people, especially women, practice yoga is to develop body strength without gaining too much weight; It is that wonderful control force in our body that helps us a lot in everyday life and keeps us slim. When we practice yoga, we usually load the joints in different asanas. These can be as light and easy as the Kumbhakasana approach, or they could be more complicated than the complete stands. However, what they have in common is the strengthening of the muscles and the weight of the bones and joints with the weight so that the tissues that make up our joints are strengthened, loosened and stabilized to promote maximum joint health.

Flexibility: Some of the anti-injury capabilities of yoga and its ability to promote joint integrity are due to the fact that it helps us increase our flexibility.

When the joints have more freedom of movement, wear is greatly reduced and can be softened and relaxed to optimize healing. Moving in repetitive patterns and, consequently, becoming stiff and tense, is one of the main causes of numerous injuries both in athletes and in normal people. Can you avoid it so easily: the secret? Do yoga!

Most people are only interested in physical and brazen aspects, such as imaginative postures, hand supports, and superhuman flexibility skills, but one of the most important reasons why yoga helps promote longevity does not. It is in strenuous postures, or when you stretch, you breathe. Yogic breathing technique is known as the art of pranayama (prana is the word used to describe universal energy or the force that surrounds us). B. K. S. Iyengar stated that "Pranayama is a conscious extension of inhalation, retention and exhalation" and he really hit the spot. It is used in various yogic yoga practices and styles to induce a meditative state and often has profound effects on energy levels and mood.

Breathing: Yogic breathing can help reduce the frequency of breathing in an individual.

The body trains to breathe more deeply and slowly, instead of breathing in the most typical, superficial, swollen and terrified way we usually do, especially in Western society. The reduction in respiratory rate can also help reduce heart rate, which in turn leads to a reduction in blood pressure and the relief of unnecessary stresses and anxiety. You can stretch your muscles more effectively if you breathe properly, deeply and slowly, which gives you many more benefits.

More efficient breathing eventually brings more oxygen to the body with less effort and, therefore, provides great rest to the heart, lungs and other organs. When they are less stressed during break time, they are at less risk of damage or wear. Yoga and yogic breathing studies have shown that they help reduce the risk of cardiovascular disorders. In addition to breathing, it has also been shown that yoga as an aerobic activity reduces the risk of heart disease. This is important when it comes to longevity because heart disease is a major cause of death in both men and women and can be prevented with a healthy routine.

Finally, yoga promotes longevity so effectively because of the profound effects it often has on the way its practitioners see their lives and bodies.

With so much emphasis on finding harmony, living the moment and experiencing the body and the self, yoga causes people to become much more aware of their body and the feelings they experience daily. When you practice yoga regularly, it is much easier to notice small things such as a slightly abnormal feeling in the stomach or a feeling of slight imbalance around the shoulder, etc. Being aware of the body all the time does a lot to ensure safety and sensitivity, helping people take care of their bodies. Being more aware of breathing and the body could surely save many people from many of the problems they have, often caused by things like overeating and living sedentary, or by going through injuries unnecessarily. Self-awareness, in many ways, is undoubtedly the best gift yoga can give many of us.

REASONS TO PRACTICE YOGA FOR HEALTH AND LONGEVITY

In the United States, many people have been reported practicing yoga for health, be it physical health, mental health, spiritual health or a combination of the three. When you look around in an American yoga studio, you are likely to see people of all shapes, sizes and ages. The study of yoga can be a different place, with people of all levels seeking a form of health in their practice. What all these people have in common is that they have discovered the yoga unique ability to promote health and life span.

THE HISTORY OF YOGA

The first recorded practice of yoga dates back thousands of years ago. The practice was based on a global philosophy of man who sought harmony with himself and with the world and, as such, was and continues to be a practice that includes breathing, meditation and exercise. Despite its long history, yoga only arrived in the United States in the 19th century.

In the United States and other Western countries, yoga has been associated primarily with the practice of asanas (also known as postures) of Hatha Yoga and is generally considered a form of exercise despite its deeper origins. While some complaint about the western marketing of yoga, many others applaud its growing popularity and accessibility.

SEVEN REASONS TO PRACTICE YOGA FOR HEALTH

Regardless of your skill level or the type of yoga you practice, yoga can work wonders for your health and wellbeing both today and tomorrow. A regular yoga practice can also slow down the negative physical effects associated with our generally sedentary lifestyles and aging. Better yet, yoga adapts to all levels and ages, which means that your body, mind and soul can benefit from yoga until old age. Here are seven excellent reasons to begin your yoga practice for a healthier life and longevity.

Mobility: A typical American yoga practice usually consists of a series of postures that take place during different periods. Many of these positions are simple but challenging and require strength and flexibility that you may not have yet. While yoga can take you to the physical limit, it can also expand it.

After just a couple of sessions, many noticed that postures become easier and more fluid as they develop their strength and flexibility, allowing them to "deepen" their posture or draw their attention to another aspect of the pose. To prevent the common complaint of aches and pains in old age, it is possible to resort to yoga to relieve the necessary pain and stretching. Maintaining your flexibility and range of movement in your older years can also keep your body healthy and improve your quality of life.

Strength and muscle tone: While yoga increases flexibility, it also increases muscle strength. Yoga makes us stronger through the sustained celebration of postures, controlled transitions, and of course, the postures themselves. More importantly, yoga involves muscles that cannot be used or strengthened daily, adding general tone and strength and even giving a vital boost to bone density.

Balance: With so many older Americans who suffer fractures and other serious health problems after an avoidable fall, it shouldn't be a problem that we should all work to maintain not only our strength and flexibility in old age but also our balance. Yoga incorporates all kinds of asanas, including several basic balancing postures, that can provide the safe balance practice we all need. With a better balance comes greater communication between the two hemispheres of the brain and a much safer way to reach our oldest years.

Weight loss: With approximately 1/3 of American adults considered overweight or obese, we need to discover a method to attack the deadly epidemic or preventing it from happening. Experts conclude that the way to achieve and maintain a healthy weight should include changes in both diet and lifestyle, including an increase in physical exercises. Yoga is free to anyone of all shapes and sizes, and the practice can help you lose weight and control a healthy weight in several ways:

Yoga enables people to be more aware of their bodies and the need to take care of themselves, including exercise and healthy eating.

Yoga can help people get a sense of control over their body and their food choices, as well as reduce the stress that often causes overeating.

Many of the asanas (postures) stimulate the glands, such as the thyroid gland, which can help increase metabolism and promote balance in the body.

Detoxification: It is said that yoga helps to detoxify the body since many of the postures stimulate blood flow to the different organs, effectively helping the body in the natural process of toxin elimination. Yoga also strongly emphasizes breathing techniques that not only provide guidance during physical practice but also greater oxygenation of the body. Some of the postures particularly stimulate the digestive tract in the stomach, which can improve digestion in our system.

Stress and Anxiety Reduction: Yoga educates us to be in the moment and to focus on ourselves and our breathing. It is said that the practice gives people a sense of control over situations and the strength and tranquillity of letting go of those things that cannot be controlled. Many call their yoga sessions therapy. It is known that the reduction of stress and relaxation associated with the practice of yoga are useful for several things, from lowering blood pressure to improving sleep quality, which can not only increase your life but can make everyone happier These years won.

Self-awareness: It is said that yoga makes people aware of their bodies, minds and emotions. However, more importantly, regular yoga practice also provides those same people with tools to help deal with the problems that arise in that self-awareness. For example, people suffering from pain may find positions that affect and relieve pain, as well as overcome feelings of helplessness.

Common Sense Warnings: Yoga can provide health benefits for almost everyone, and you should always consult your doctor before starting a new exercise routine. People with the conditions below should consult their doctor before beginning a yoga practice:

    i.   High blood pressure

    ii.   Risk of blood clots

    iii.   Eye conditions, including glaucoma

    iv.   osteoporosis

12 REASONS WHY YOGA HELPS IMPROVE THE LIFESPAN

Whether you practice yoga daily or have followed your first yoga class, you have probably noticed some benefits: relaxed mood, better sleep or more energy. Although we are still learning and measuring the benefits of yoga, Western science is discovering clues about this ancient practice and influencing longevity and life span. These are only 12 of the many benefits that influence longevity and promote long and healthy life.

1. Prevents cartilage and joint breakage: Yoga takes the joints through its full range of movements, which helps the articular cartilage to receive fresh nutrients, prevents wear and protects the bones. That also helps prevent arthritis from degenerate.

2. Increases bone strength and density: Different postures in yoga require weight-bearing, which strengthens the bones and helps prevent osteoporosis. Specifically, yoga strengthens the bones of the arm, particularly vulnerable to osteoporotic fractures. Many studies have shown that the practice of yoga increases bone density in general.

3. Increase blood flow: Yoga makes the blood flow! The relaxation helps the circulation, the movement brings more oxygen to the cells (which works best as a result), the torsion brings fresh oxygenated blood to the organs and the investments reverse the blood flow from the lower part of the body to the brain and the heart. Besides, yoga increases hemoglobin levels in red blood cells, which helps prevent blood clots, heart attacks and strokes.

4. Cleans lymph and immune system: Yoga movements help drain the lymph, allowing the system to better combat the inflection, destroy diseased cells and release toxic waste in the body. Also, meditation have a beneficial effect on the functioning of the immune system, increasing it when necessary (that is, increasing antibody levels in response to a vaccine) and decreasing it when necessary (that is, aggressively mitigating an inappropriate immune function aggressively in an autoimmune disease such as psoriasis).

5. Increase your heart rate: Many lessons like power yoga can increase heart rate in the aerobic range. Studies have found that yoga can reduce resting heart rate, increase endurance and improve maximum oxygen absorption during physical activity, all reflecting better aerobic atmosphere. Studies have also found that those who practice pranayama or "breath control" can exercise more with less oxygen. Moving your heart rate regularly in the aerobic range reduces the risk of heart attack and can relieve depression.

6. It regulates the adrenal glands: Yoga reduces cortisol levels. If they are elevated, they compromise the immune system and can lead to permanent changes in the brain. Excess cortisol has also been associated with major depression, osteoporosis, hypertension and insulin resistance.

7. Lower blood sugar: Yoga lowers blood sugar and LDL ("bad") cholesterol and increases HDL ("good") cholesterol. In people with diabetes, yoga has been found to reduce blood sugar by reducing cortisol and adrenaline levels, encouraging weight loss and improving sensitivity to the effects of insulin. Reducing blood sugar levels reduces the risk of diabetic complications, such as heart attack, kidney failure and blindness.

8. Improve your balance: Practicing yoga regularly increases proprioception (the ability to feel what your body is doing and where it is in space) and improves balance. A better balance could mean fewer falls. For the elderly, this translates into greater independence and a delay in admission to a nursing home or never entering it.

9. Relaxes the nervous system and assists you sleep better: Stimulations and activities in our modern society can tax our nervous system. Yoga and meditation encourage the inversion of the senses and the elimination of stimuli, providing the necessary downtime of the nervous system and better sleep, which means that you will be less tired, stressed and less prone to accidents.

10. Allow the lung to breathe properly: Yogis sometimes take fewer breaths of large volume, which is soothing and very relaxing. Yoga breathing technique has been shown to help people with lung problems due to congestive insufficiency and improve lung function measurements, including maximum breathing volume and expiration efficiency. Yoga encourages breathing through the nose, which filters, heats, and moistens the air. That helps prevent asthma attacks, also eliminates pollen, dirt, and other things that you would rather not take in the lungs.

11. Better digestion: Yoga promotes healthy digestion by moving the body in a way that facilitates the faster and more efficient transport of food and waste products through the intestines. Healthy digestion helps reduce the risk of colon cancer and diseases of the digestive tract.

12. Promotes self-care and a healthy lifestyle: Perhaps the greatest benefits of yoga are its ability to inspire and improve self-care and healthy life. Because yogis tend to be more involved in their health and care, they discover they have the power to make positive changes in their lives and adopt healthier habits. Over time, a healthy lifestyle has a great impact on life expectancy.

CHAPTER EIGHT

BREATHE FOR BETTER LONGEVITY

How to breathe, breathing tips, breathing instructions, yoga breathing

Only a few of us have cultivated good breathing habits and most of us will never know if we do not participate in yoga or breathing sessions. Good breathing habits can make your body more productive and effective, both in and out of training, and have the added advantages of preventing the stress effect. Here are some helpful tips and exercises to help you get the most out of each breath.

Suggestion 1: the lower lungs are better breaths

If you see a child breathing, you can see the slow rise of the abdomen during inhalation and the slight softening of the abdomen during exhalation. That is called diaphragmatic breathing. However, at some point, many of us lose this natural breathing pattern. We begin to pull the belly by inhalation, forcing the air into the upper lobes of the lungs. From a scientific point of view, "thoracic respiration is inefficient because the highest amount of blood flow occurs in the lower lobes of the lungs... Rapid and superficial breathing in the chest translates into less oxygen transfer to the blood and, consequently, bad delivery of nutrients to the tissues in the body. If you train your body to breathe in the lower lungs, you may notice that you can maintain physical exercise, as well as daily life, with less effort.

Suggestion 2: breathing indicates awareness

There is no natural and unconscious movement model for the body. For this reason, it is entirely possible to learn a movement, such as running, cycling or yoga, and repeat it with little or no awareness. However, if we stop paying attention to breathing, our unconscious rhythm will take action. Therefore, it is easy to know if we are present in a breathing yoga class, and this practice can move to many areas of our lives. Our breathing indicates our level of awareness and presence in each situation.

Suggestion 3: we can change our unconscious breathing pattern

Ideally, we would like to reach a point where, even when we stop paying attention, the breath regains its natural pattern. We do this by training the breath, as we do with the body, through constant practice. Try this exercise to experience deep and diaphragmatic breathing:

Lying on your back, put one hand on your belly and another on your heart.

Exhale all the air in your lungs.

Inhale and breathe only in the belly. You feel it rises in your hand. Exhale your belly. Do it three times.

On the next inhalation, breathe only in the ribs, the point between the two hands. Feel the ribs expand up, down and in all directions. Exhale the ribs. Do it three times.

On the next inhalation, breathe only in the heart space at the top of the chest. He feels that he is facing his chin. Exhale the heart. Do it three times.

On the next inhalation, breathe a third of the breath in the abdomen, a third of the breath in the ribs and a third of the breath in the heart space. Exhale first from the heart, then from the ribs, then from the belly. Do it three times too. This practice will help you feel what it is like to start breathing from below and exercise. It's amazing how much controls you have over your body which help you to send your breath to different points of the lungs and ribs.

Suggestion 4: diaphragmatic breathing increases lung capacity

It is believed that we can inhale up to two liters of air in a single breath. Many of us probably only use a small amount of that ability, which makes us breathe more than necessary. Each breath is a use of our energy, and therefore, being more effective with breathing, we waste less energy. When the diaphragm is pressed against the ribs, there is less room for breathing. When the diaphragm first moves away from the ribs, it opens the space and creates a vacuum effect, pushing the air towards the base of the ribs. Here, the lungs are effective and we get the added benefit of breathing more in general.

Suggestion 5: diaphragmatic breathing reduces stress

Of all the reasons why people come to my yoga class, stress reduction is among the top three. I think we all know someone who takes care of too much stress and even someone could be you. If you are looking for a simple and free way to reduce stress, look no further than diaphragmatic breathing. When we breathe in this way, we can reduce our heart rate and possibly our blood pressure. These are two key signals to the brain that all is well with our body. In fact, slow breathing in itself tells the brain that we are doing well, causing the brain to release fewer stress hormones from our endocrine system. That also gives the body the possibility of activating the parasympathetic nervous system, essentially intervening and reversing the effects of the stress hormones already present in the body.

Yogis have long known that breathing is the connection between the outer world and the inner world. We use the same word, prana, to describe breath, energy and life itself. Whenever you think about it, pay attention to your breathing. If you spend a day when you have not consciously thought about your breathing, it could cause more stress subconsciously in a way that can be easily resolved for the benefit of your health and longevity.

LONGEVITY RESISTANCE

Good breathing habits are widely considered essential components of health. Unfortunately, many people take shallow breaths, use only part of their lungs and often hold their breath when they get nervous or tense.

Breathing well is vital to your health. Bruce Frantzis taught us this system, who says that if you ever do one thing to improve your health, learning to breathe well would be the best option.

The basic techniques of respiratory longevity ensure that everything inside your body moves and synchronizes with the rhythm of your breathing. The diligent practice of this breathing technique cultivates good health, the ability to relax at any time and concentrate for long periods.

LONGEVITY BREATHING

Longevity breathing removes carbon dioxide and increases the usable oxygen that is inhaled. Even if you can inhale enough to attract enough oxygen to your system, you may not exhale deeply or enough to get rid of all the carbon dioxide in your body. For most people, about a quarter of the reserve in the lower part of the lungs is always full of carbon dioxide.

This leaves only three-quarters of the lungs free for oxygen intake at the next inhalation. It causes the exhalation to weaken further, decreasing the body's ability to provide oxygen from the air. Breathing improperly:

DECREASE OXYGEN CONSUMPTION

It causes the accumulation of toxic waste in the blood, which often causes yawning.

Reduces mental capacity and clarity and increases stress in the body. It also Increases the accumulated carbon dioxide.

Respiratory longevity helps you create and stabilize a constant breathing pattern that mitigates excessive emotional oscillations. Improve your nervous system to relax and make your thoughts more fluid and more comfortable. Studying your breathing patterns can make you aware of how your moods and emotions change.

For example, fear tends to produce irregular and tired breathing or to hold your breath without realizing it, this is part of a reaction to stress and tends to increase its severity. Shallow breathing makes people prone to lung weakness against environmental problems, such as polluted air, and can even lead to depression.

According to traditional Chinese medicine, the ability of your breathing to improve the functioning of internal organs (liver, kidneys, heart, spleen and lungs) is as valuable as increasing your oxygen consumption. Longevity breathing methods transfer the pressure of the air entering the lungs to internal organs, particularly the heart. This provides a smooth but firm massage to the organs, increasing blood flow and helping others optimize their natural range of movements.

When the range of movement of the internal organs decreases, blood flow to the internal organs also decreases, blocking the regular flow of energy. Other effects include gradual shortening of the ligaments and limited movement of the organs. Body functions will gradually weaken and eventually, the disease will hit

BREATHING EXERCISE FOR HEALING AND LONGEVITY

At this point in this book, we will discuss a healing breathing exercise that will prolong your life and lead to advanced healing for any pre-existing health condition in the body.

Breathing exercise improves circulation, thanks to a process called vasodilation, which helps the growth of new blood vessels. That can also increase the production of more capillaries between veins and arteries.

Its capillaries are an essential part of the circulatory system and the distribution of oxygen and carbon dioxide throughout the body. This increase in the production of capillaries, therefore, allows a much more efficient use of the levels of O2 and CO2 inside the body, improving the general circulation within the body. This improves the overall efficiency or ability of your heart to pump blood throughout the system.

How this affects endurance and overall sports performance

If you are an athlete, or simply want to improve your overall level of fitness and endurance, this breathing exercise for healing and longevity is also excellent for this. When general circulation and blood flow is improved, combined with the production of more red blood cells and new blood vessels, we now have greater overall functionality and higher levels of athletic endurance at our disposal.

How does this breathing exercise result in an anti-aging?

One of the essential aspects of this breathing exercise for healing and longevity is the way in which it actively releases stem cells in the body. We actively release stem cells through an induced state of intermittent hypoxia that causes low levels of oxygen in the blood.

Russian doctors have investigated this particular hypoxic state for decades. They also studied the effects it has on professional athletes and their ability to perform at higher levels. Yogis also knew the benefits of creating this state within the body. They have been practicing it for thousands of years.

How can we stimulate stem cells and cell repair with this breathing exercise for healing and longevity?

When stem cells are released in the body, they can flow where they are most needed. Stem cells have this extraordinary ability to adapt to transform and grow in any other cell in the body. This is why much research is currently being done on stem cells and how they can be used to treat, regenerate and grow new tissues.

We are not only able to naturally release these stem cells in the body, but we can also point to particular positions within the body through the act of intention and concentration. By using this breathing exercise we can concentrate our intention and even contract the muscles in the area that we want to recover. It tells the body to move the stem cells to that specific position. It can be a potent process of self-healing and understand how to work with your body at deeper levels.

How does this healing breathing exercise affect the overall health of the brain?

When general blood flow is improved along with a much more efficient O_2-CO_2 exchange, it has naturally improved functionality within all other organs of the body. One of the largest organs that seem to be affected by this is your brain. This is simply because your brain tends to use a lot of oxygen regularly. This additional efficiency of the use of oxygen within the body can also lead to the activation of latent parts of the brain, as well as improve cognitive function and memory.

CHAPTER NINE

LEARN TO SMILE MORE FOR HEALTH, HAPPINESS, YOUNG LOOK AND LONGEVITY

Happiness makes life enjoyable can also lead to better health, well-being and longevity. To get the most out of life and get started, try the smile skills described below. To test its potency, try it for a week. Consider it a smiling one week experiment. If you commit to following these simple steps to smile more, you will be on your way to living a happier and healthier life.

Steps to happiness

What you will do: throughout the week, you will concentrate on smiling more. You will develop a way to remind yourself to smile during the day and even force a smile on your face from time to time. Why? Research shows that smiling improves your mood and makes you become more positive.

How does it works: Medical researchers think that by forcing a smile, a specific set of facial muscles is activated. That set of muscles is closely related to the emotions of happiness and joy. Smiling, you tell the emotional centers of your brain to tell them that everything is fine. Then, even if it isn't, it will be soon.

Motivate yourself: smiling more is an easy way to gradually develop the quality of your life and increase longevity. All you need to become ever young is to smile and you will become a happier person. Really. It's that easy.

Ways to smile more

The smile is the natural response to something fun, happy or fun, so it is apparent that you probably do not need help with the automatic smile response. To learn to smile more, you must first practice:

Practice smiling: SMILE! Do it now while reading this book. Put a big warm smile on that face of yours. It is not a fake, strange smile, but a real smile, as if you had seen a long-time friend after many years of absence. Now, think of something opposite, but keep smiling. It's hard to keep an unhappy or negative thought in your mind while keeping a smile on your face. The smile can help increase happiness and decrease negativity.

Give yourself a smile: Now that you have practiced a smile and have understood a little about how the smile can improve your mood, the trick is to remember to smile always. You will probably need a reminder to smile often. Choose something you feel, see or often do during the day to be your "smile signal." You can choose a sound as a reminder, such as a ringing phone or an email notification tone. You can choose an action, such as getting in or out of the car, to remind you to smile. You can choose a visual reminder, such as seeing someone drinking coffee or seeing someone laugh. Challenge yourself to smile every time you follow your signals throughout the week.

Stay motivated: people who smile while talking make a much better impression because they seem safer and friendlier. You can even "hear" a smile on the phone. If you smile during a call, the tone of your voice will be cleared and you can establish a better connection through the phone.

TIPS TO SMILE MORE

While steps 1 to 3 above provide everything you need to challenge yourself to smile more, here are some other tips to help you:

Do not look strange. Make your smiles natural, warm and sincere. You are merely trying to maintain a good mood. Even a small, almost imperceptible smile can alter your mood.

Smile when you think about it, not only when you encounter the smile signal. Think of something you really like when you smile: it will help you make your smile sincere. Think about your favorite vacation spot, driving a new car or a good friend. Take a deep breath while smiling. This will help reduce the stress you have and give you a moment to enjoy your smile. One or two deep breaths increase relaxation and improve your mood.

CAN TAKING NAPS IMPACT LONGEVITY?

Scientists have not yet figured out why we sleep, but they know that this daily ritual is crucial for long and healthier life. In addition, research has consistently shown that people who suffer from shuteye in both quality and quantity are less sensitive to serious illnesses such as heart disease, high blood pressure, diabetes and obesity. Curious to know exactly how sleep affects longevity? Here are some explanations.

SLEEP AND THE IMMUNE SYSTEM

Most of us know the effects that bad sleep has on us the next day: we are sleepy, our memory banks do not work as well and we struggle to perform mental and even routine physical tasks. However, we rarely notice the long-term effects and the impact on our longevity because they are minute and we have become accustomed to poor sleeping habit. Slowly we compress the pounds and suffer more from common colds and the flu without connecting our bad sleeping habits with our growing number of ailments. Sleep quality has long been related to weight and the immune system. Research has shown that less sleep alters the metabolic pathways that regulate appetite; We end up feeling more hungry as a result.

There is a higher chance that we may get sick. A recent study by scientists from the Internal Medicine Archive found that, of the 153 men and women who participated, those who slept on average less than seven hours a night were three times more likely to get sick than those who had an average of at least eight hours.

How can sleep affect our lives for longer? Many experts believe that sleep offers the brain the ability to recharge and optimize the functions of our body. Dr. Michael Twery, who is National Centre for Research's director on Sleep Disorders, states that a region of the brain known as the suprachiasmatic nucleus orchestrates hormones and other changes throughout the body effective preparation of sleep.

 By keeping this system aligned, falling asleep when our bodies signal us to do so, we are optimizing our rates of metabolism and cardiovascular systems, among other functions, within our body system. However, if we are struggling with a sleep disorder, estimated between 50 and 70 million Americans, we are not letting our bodies do their best. This eventually puts us at risk of more serious diseases that affect our longevity.

REM: OUR UNKNOWN HERO FROM OUR BRAIN: Sleeping well at night is measured not only by how much we sleep, but also by how well we sleep. In fact, the deepest phase of sleep, which is the REM phase, is the unknown hero of the brain, since this is where the most intense neuronal activity occurs: it increases blood circulation and oxygen levels. Furthermore, our brain tissue absorbs more amino acids. Scientists say that this is the reason why those who sleep well are not only acute thinkers, but also have less risk of neurological diseases along the way, especially Alzheimer's disease.

DEEP SLUMBER = BEAUTY DREAM: Not surprisingly, the sleeping beauty looked so young after sleeping for 100 years. While we sleep, the free radicals responsible for premature aging are destroyed. After a good night's sleep, we seem rejuvenated and renewed.

In addition, the body's cells are more productive during deep sleep when there is a reduction in protein degradation. Proteins are considered the basic components of our body: they have the task of creating more cells and repairing skin damage due to sun exposure and stress. This means that any recent skin damage will be repaired during this period.

SLEEP WELL DURING YOUR GOLDEN YEARS: Many of us believe we need less sleep as we get older. This is true for most stages of life: 16-18 hours for new-borns, 10-12 hours for young children, nine hours for older children and teenagers, and seven to eight hours for adults. However, the elderly need to sleep as much as teenagers. Older people who sleep nine or more hours are more likely to enjoy their golden years and live longer.

Unfortunately, the aging process can make our sleep difficult. For instance, the hormone melatonin helps set the body's sleep clock, but its levels slowly decrease with age. In fact, it's been found by different research that some older adults produce minimal or no amounts. Natural melatonin supplements can counteract this effect. Although the aging process is inevitable for all of us, we can delay it by sleeping optimally every night, paving the way for us to look younger, feel better and, ultimately, live longer.

CHAPTER TEN

SKINCARE AND SKIN PHYSIOLOGY

The skin, which is the largest organ of the human body protects our bodies from the harsh environment, maintains body temperature, expels waste, provides sensory information to the brain and regulates body moisture. We think of our skin more than any other part of our body and show so much attention by investing our emotions and about 6-20% of our disposable income in our skin (Lappe, 1996). It is worth considering, therefore, how cosmetic products affect our skin. In this book, we will examine the psychosocial impact of cosmetics and why cosmetics are considered necessary. The physiology of the skin, how cosmetics influence the function of the skin and the effects of synthetic and natural cosmetic ingredients on the skin will also be considered.

The psychosocial impact of cosmetics

Our society is concerned with the "culture of beauty" (Lappe, 1996) that includes the idea that our skin should always look young and free from imperfections. Our psychological well-being is often closely related to the perceptions of how our skin looks before ourselves and others. We define our own image to include the visible representation of our skin before others, so it has become the "main canvas on which our cultural and personal identity is drawn" (Lappe, 1996). Cosmetic companies neglect the concepts of natural beauty to highlight defects such as large pores, fine lines and wrinkles, which influence our spending habits in the search for the perfect skin condition.

In the animal kingdom, most of the male species are endowed with colored physical attributes so that a less colored but wisely camouflaged female partner is attracted to it. Humans have no equivalent ornaments, so women use cosmetics, especially makeup, to decorate their faces to attract potential partners.

The need for cosmetics

A cosmetic is any substance that, when applied, causes a temporary and superficial change (Anctzak, 2001). We use a lot of cosmetics on our skin, from moisturizers to lipstick. Makeup alters our visual appearance by improving and perfecting our facial features through the artistic application of color of different types and tones. It can beautify the face, which also helps to express our sense of identity to others. Makeup can hide imperfections, scars, dark circles, or even skin tone. It can increase self-esteem, make us feel more attractive and increase our social acceptability in some social situations. The use of makeup can contribute to a well-maintained image, which positively influences our confidence, self-esteem, health and morals.

Skincare cosmetics treat the upmost surface layer of the skin by providing the best protection and aid against the environmental factors than untreated skin. Creams treat the surface of the skin by imparting moisture to the skin cells in the outermost layer of the skin. It also forms a thin barrier that traps the underlying moisture, thus preventing water from evaporating from the skin's surface. Creams also speed the hydration of skin cells in the outer layer, giving the skin a temporarily smooth and plump appearance. The scrubs improve the appearance of the skin by removing scaly skin, blackheads, and some dead cells. The astringent enhances the tone and texture of the skin by inflating the walls of the pores so that dirt and debris do not accumulate inside. Soaps loosen dirt and grime books by dissolving the remaining fat in the skin of oils, natural creams and makeup.

THE PHYSIOLOGICAL CONCEPT OF THE SKIN AND HOW COSMETICS AFFECT THE FUNCTION OF THE SKIN

The skin is composed of three main layers which are the epidermis, the dermis, and the hypodermis. The epidermis is the only layer out of the three we can see with our eyes and as we age, there are notable changes that are hidden from our eyes. For example, the skin gradually becomes thinner over time, especially around the eyes. Some cosmeceuticals may slightly thicken the skin, but the thinning process is inevitable. Elastin and collagen, located in the dermis region of the skin, keep the skin elastic and hydrated, but with aging, these fibers break to form lines and wrinkles. The exposure to ultraviolet radiation accelerates this process and, since few cosmetics can reach the dermis, the idea that a cosmetic can reverse this process is unfounded. The best way to prevent wrinkles and wrinkles is to limit our exposure to the sun and ultraviolet radiation.

The skin is complex and has a very dynamic tissue system. A square inch of skin is made up of 19 million cells, 625 sweat glands, 90 sebaceous glands, 65 hair follicles, 19,000 sensory cells, and 4 meters of blood vessels. The outermost layer of the epidermis section of the is called the cornified layer and consists of keratin sheets, a protein, and scales, dead and flat skin cells. It is our barrier against dehydration of the environment. It receives its main moisture input from the underlying tissue since constant contact with the external environment tends to dry the skin's surface. When the skin is opened to dry conditions, the cornified layer can become dry, brittle, hard, and if left untreated, can break and cause infection. Creams generate a waxy barrier to prevent dehydration and keep skin moist and elastic. Under the cornified layer, there are six other layers of the epidermis responsible for cell generation. The life cycle of the skin cells in this layer lasts approximately 28 days, so it can take three to four weeks to observe any change in the surface of the skin by the use of a new cosmetic.

The skin's surface also harbors millions of healthy microorganisms that increase our immunity to pathogenic bacteria or cause diseases. Therefore, in out attempt to sterilize the skin, we also destroys beneficial bacteria, such as mutant streptococcus and the luteal micrococcus. Toners, for example, are useful for containing bacterial populations, thereby reducing acne exacerbations resulting from microbes that invade and proliferate in the pores. Excessive use of antimicrobial agents can produce harmful results when too many beneficial bacteria are destroyed, allowing pathogenic bacteria to multiply without control over the skin. The skin produces antimicrobial proteins, two of which are called defensins and cathelicidins, which advances when the skin is damaged. Perspiration is necessary to maintain the internal temperature of the body. It also expels a germicidal protein called dermcidin to fight the bacteria that produce body odor. Deodorants also help keep the bacterial population low, thereby reducing odors produced while feeding on debris expelled from the sweat glands. Research has shown that people who wash in excess are more prone to infections and eczema due to the "washing" of natural bacteria and germicides too often.

EFFECTS OF NATURAL AND SYNTHETIC COSMETIC INGREDIENTS ON THE SKIN According to Antczak, 2001, the natural substance is said to be any plant or animal extract, rock, or mineral that is obtained from the earth while an artificial or synthetic substance is a substance that has been modified by chemical reactions in an industrial process. We use a lot of cosmetics on our skin, but before using these beauty products, three essential questions must be asked:

- What is the composition of the cosmetic?

- Why is each ingredient used?

- Do the ingredients have positive or negative effects on the skin and body?

Many products claim to be very safe or even appear safe, but in addition to the short-term benefits of using the cosmetic, are there long-term effects as a result of the daily absorption of its use? The skin was considered an impermeable barrier, but transdermal drugs have shown that the opposite is true; The skin allows many substances to pass through its layers into the bloodstream.

Several factors influence the speed at which the skin will absorb various cosmetic ingredients. Skin conditions, for example, if it is dry or damaged, increase absorption. Even cuts, acne, or abrasions increase absorption. Other ways to absorb cosmetic ingredients are to inhale them, for example, with hairspray or talcum powder or through mucous membranes. Wet substances are absorbed more easily and the skinless absorb dust. Many products claim to cure skin problems, such as acne or dry skin but what you discover is that they contain ingredients that aggravate these problems that they claim to cure. For example, acne treatments may contain comedogenic ingredients or block pores. Creams that should treat dry skin can actually take away from the skin its natural oils that are useful for preventing dryness. Some contain chemicals that penetrate the skin and dissolve skin oils and degrease the skin. A growing trend is a chemical sensitivity that can develop at any time, even after long-term use of the same product. The ingredients of many cosmetics make 20% of the population (data from the USA, Erickson, 2002) develop symptoms of chemical sensitivity. Natural cosmetics emphasizes the most traditional skin treatments with few of these severe effects, recognizing that short-term beauty does not compensate for long-term health risks.

The health of the skin depends on solid nutritional practices, healthy living and effective and safe protection on its surface. Organic makeup co. It can help you get healthy and radiant skin, offering a complete line of cosmetics and makeup made up of all natural ingredients, without animal, synthetic, or petroleum-derived ingredients. Once you have received your order, our products are fresh for you and contain preservatives such as d-alpha-tocopherol (vitamin E), ascorbic acid (vitamin C), and other vegetable oils with antimicrobial properties.

DRY SKIN CARE: TIPS TO IMPROVE DRY SKIN

As normal basic skincare, dry skincare should be performed daily. Proper cleaning, toning, and hydration practices should become natural and routine for your days, such as regular exercise, a healthy diet, work, and rest.

Dry skin comes from a low level of skin oil or sebum

This condition can be inherited, but many other factors can interfere with sebum production. Extreme temperatures, wind, and air conditioning can exacerbate the condition, making the skin feel tense, cracked, or cracked. Smoking, chemicals, environmental pollution, and high stress compromise dry skin and make the skin look dull and wrinkled, particularly around the eyes and mouth. One more reason to practice intelligent care of dry skin.

Skin disorders, which may include; eczema, psoriasis, dermatitis, and seborrhea, as well as some medications (such as antihistamines, antispasmodics, and diuretics), can also cause dry skin. Treating these disorders and avoiding these medications will help improve dry skin conditions.

Avoid what will make you unhealthy inside and at the same, ensure you avoid any product that can increase your chances of developing unhealthy skin or skin cancer.

Are you a smoker? I want you to imagine a day without smoking a cigarette. So imagine that you have dry, wrinkled skin that makes you look 20-30 years older than you. Is it an incentive to quit smoking and regularly take care of dry skin?

We are not saying that change is easy. But the long-term change could be the best thing that happened to you. Proper skincare in general and dry skincare, in particular, are undoubtedly available to anyone concerned with the health and appearance of their skin. Think about how you want to look and feel in six months, one year, or even two years. It can improve the appearance and feeling in a short time. Why not decide to help you get better skin?

Another thing you should quite if you want to take delight in a more healthier skin condition. This applies not only to the people with a dry skin condition but to anyone else who prefers to have smooth and beautiful skin. The number one enemy to your skin is the sun You can treat dry skin with the following tips:

PROTECT YOUR SKIN FROM THE SUN

Although many of us love the sun and love to cook in it, we walk and play with it, and we love the way it turns our skin and makes us feel healthy, agile, sexy and carefree, makes no mistake, the sun can kill you If you let me do it.

The sun gives life and provides us with essential vitamin D, but it can also cause irreversible damage to our skin, causing it to age prematurely, drying, wrinkling, diminishing and, what is more alarming, developing precancerous moles, sunspots and carcinomas, and melanomas cancerous

As much as we like the sun, we must interact with it intelligently. Here are 14 ways to improve your skin for more information on how to protect yourself from the harmful effects of excessive sun exposure.

Here are some solid tips for treating dry skincare:

In winter, when the air humidity is low, the skin dries faster. Keep this in mind when choosing a moisturizer.

Use a stronger moisturizer in winter and a lighter moisturizer in summer when the humidity is high.

As we age, our skin becomes thinner, wrinkled, and drier with time. As a result, our skin is more susceptible to damage in the form of cuts and cracks. Pay special attention when handling tools and utensils and when coming into contact with abrasive surfaces.

Exercise regularly to improve blood circulation, which helps nourish the skin and purify it from the inside.

Simple dry skincare: drink plenty of clean water to improve skin hydration. At least two rooms every day.

Thoroughly clean the skin. Because dry skin is damaged more easily than usual or oily skin, it cleans well to prevent dead cells from mixing with dirt and dirt and causing infections.

Avoid intense washing, especially with hot water, which evaporates faster than warm or lukewarm water. Excessive contact with water eliminates natural oils and skin moisture and promotes greater drying. People with dry skin conditions, especially the elderly, should avoid taking their bathing or showering with hot water.

Keep baths or showers less than 15 minutes to prevent the loss of natural oils that help retain moisture from the skin.

Avoid commercial soaps that dry the skin. Select a naturally moisturizing soap that has a moderate pH value.

Techniques for treating dry skin: after showering, gently apply virgin coconut oil on the face and gently massage to circulate the blood and refresh the face.

Avoid cold cleaning creams based on hydrogenated oils. These oils actually dry the skin and cause wrinkles. Instead, try drying virgin coconut oil or pure olive oil on your skin to purify it. Wash with warm or warm water and dry with a soft cloth.

Always moisten the skin (face, neck, body) after a bath or shower. Hydrate your hands after washing them.

Get evening primrose oil supplements to strengthen the skin and increase the moisture content of the skin. Have adequate sleep to allow the skin to repair itself at the cellular level.

 To get some fantastic ways to improve the appearance and feel of your dry skin, use simple and inexpensive products that you can buy at your local food market or at a grocery store.

 There is no mystery for proper care of dry skin. First, make the decision always to practice regular and consistent skincare. This may mean giving up something (something that probably hurts anyway) or taking all the necessary steps to promote your general physical and mental health and the health and appearance of your skin. Once you are committed to giving your skin a pleasant appearance, use common sense. Consider the guide and the previous tips for practicing proper care of dry skin and enjoying healthy and better skin for the rest of your life!

Dry skin lotion: what to do and what not to do when selecting one for the skin

Here is an effortless way to find the best lotion for dry skin. Not many people pay attention to the basics of skincare and that is why they end up using a product, which does more harm than good.

What follows in this book is a set of things to do and disregard when selecting a lotion for dry skin. If you follow them, you will surely end up buying the best and most effective skincare product.

1 - Verify the expiration date

Always verify the duration of the product you intend to use. Sometimes, we end up purchasing products that are close to their expiration date; in these cases, they not only become ineffective but can also pose a danger to the skin.

2 - Read the ingredient list

This list is a repository of product information. You can use it to your advantage and select the best lotion for dry skin. Read this list and pay attention to the harmful chemicals in the product. Any chemical compound that you don't understand is not good for you. Always keep in mind that a good quality product has simple and natural ingredients.

3 - Use natural products

The best skincare products have natural ingredients such as avocado oil, grapeseed oil, fruit extracts, algae, plants, and trees. These ingredients are useful because they attack the main cause of skin imperfections. They also nourish the skin by providing the necessary nutrients such as vitamins A, D, K, and E.

Now that you know the essentials when choosing a skin lotion, it's time to see what not to do.

What not to do

1 - Do not buy a product with alcohol

Many creams and lotions have alcohol as part of its ingredient. Alcohol by nature causes dehydration to the skin and makes it drier which extracts the moisture from the skin and makes it prone to wrinkles.

2 - Avoid scented products

I.Perfumes composed chemical substances, which are irritants, neurotoxins, and phthalates. They represent a danger to the endocrine system and the body's reproductive system. Avoid scented products at all costs.

3 - Avoid parabens

This ingredient that sounds harmless is the leading cause of many types of cancer. Many cases have been traced to the long-term use of products connected to Paraben. In fact, many countries have banned the use of parabens in skincare products.

A good and effective lotion for dry skin is natural and does not contain harmful chemicals. If you understand this fact and follow it endlessly, then there is no reason why you will ever have skin problems.

So, get up and learn more about the natural lotion for dry skin, you will be pleasantly surprised to see the amazing results of natural products.

HOW TO STIMULATE NATURAL COLLAGEN AND STAY YOUNG

To maintain firmness, our skin requires continuous production of collagen, the protein responsible for skin firmness. However, the production of such proteins decreases when we are 30 years old. That can lead to the relaxation of the skin, which could contribute to the early emergence of wrinkles. To overcome that, natural collagen must be stimulated to reproduce at a level that maintains firmness.

This only indicates that our skin will need collagen, so the perfect way to deal with this problem is to feed it with collagen. It is sad to say that we cannot use a skin cream that contains collagen to increase its presence because soluble collagen molecules are too large and cannot be absorbed through the skin. What we need is natural collagen that can effectively contribute to the firmness and ensure that our skin looks younger.

Therefore, we look for natural compounds that can stimulate the production of natural collagen. One of these ingredients features functional keratin made from New Zealand sheep wool. This compound has been clinically proven to stimulate collagen re-growth successfully.

This compound has a partner that also helps stimulate the skin to reproduce this protein and is called Nano-Lipobelle H EQ10. It is a unique form of "nanoemulsion" so it can penetrate deep into the skin. Many studies have shown that it can provide an anti-wrinkle effect, which can be equated with young-looking skin, due to its ability to increase the production of collagen in the skin.

Natural collagen is not the only one that helps you get younger skin. Another skin protein that must be credited for its important role in maintaining skin elasticity is elastin. These two proteins work together to ensure that our skin stays young and has no wrinkles.

But maintaining that skin cannot be achieved without the help of ingredients that contain moisturizing properties. These natural ingredients are active Manuka honey, which acts to restore and rejuvenate the skin to make it softer and younger, and grapeseed oil, which moisturizes and reduces stretch marks on the skin. It contains linolenic acid and essential oils necessary for healthy skin.

A GUIDE TO THE BEST NATURAL SKINCARE PRODUCT

Let me ask you a simple question. Do you know what skincare products you currently use contain? You may not realize that the current product could cause long-term damage.

Decide to get more information and discover for yourself the best natural skincare product on the market today. Forget celebrity announcements and outrageous claims and dig a little deeper to discover what makes a product excellent and potentially harmful.

Traditional ingredients

Many of the ingredients used today in the most popular products have been used for years without any problems and, recent reports suggest that some of these ingredients could cause damage.

Parabens have been used successfully as preservatives for many years, but now they are in the spotlight as recent reports have shown that they are present in tumors taken from patients with breast cancer. Although there is no evidence that parabens are part of the cause of this form of cancer, the fact that they are connected is worrisome.

Many products contain mineral oils as a moisturizing ingredient. These are petroleum by-products that cover the skin to help retain moisture. However, they clog pores and interfere with the skin's natural abilities to eliminate toxins. This interference can cause imperfections, pimples, and could promote acne. The natural oil of the skin is taken away, which results in dryness, cracking, and premature aging.

Under the term fragrance, more than 4,000 different substances are collected. It is already known that some of these are toxic or carcinogenic and yet they are still included in skincare products.

In one of the known products, there are more than 50 different ingredients, 14 of which could be potentially harmful. This information alone was enough to want to learn more about natural skincare products.

Natural ingredients

Natural skincare is nothing new, in fact, it is older than you think. More than 3000 years ago, in ancient Egypt, Cleopatra was known for her beauty regime, and the ancient Greeks used honey for its exceptional healing and restorative qualities.

Honey continues to play an important role in natural skincare, and science has now revealed its incredible antibacterial powers. Active manuka honey is one of the most powerful honey and has been used to help heal wounds and relieve skin disorders.

Grapeseed oil is used to place a protective film on the skin to retain moisture without clogging pores and repel dirt from everyday life. It contains natural vitamin E and linoleic acid that is essential for healthy skin.

Cynergy TK (TM) is a New Zealand sheep wool extract that has extraordinary restorative capabilities. It has been revealed in clinical studies that it stimulates the new growth of skin cells and stimulates the production of collagen and elastin in the skin.

For every potentially harmful traditional ingredient, there is an effective natural alternative. If using the best natural skincare product is something that interests you, visit my website for more information. You'll be glad you did.

IS LONGEVITY DETERMINED BY GENETICS?

Human life is influenced by genetics, environment, and lifestyle. Environmental improvements since 1900 have significantly lengthened the average lifespan with significant improvements in the availability of food and clean water, better housing and housing conditions, reduced exposure to infectious diseases and access to medical care. The most important factors were advances in public health that reduced premature death by reducing the risk of infant mortality, increasing the chances of surviving childhood and avoiding infections and communicable diseases. Now people in the United States live on average around 80 years, but some survive for much longer.

Scientists are studying people in their ninety years (called nonagenarians) and hundreds (called centenarians, including semi-supercentenarians 105-109 years and supercentenarians, over 110 years old) to determine what contributes to their long life. They discovered that long-term people have little in common in education, income, or profession. However, the similarities they share reflect their lifestyle: many are not smokers, are not obese and cope well with stress. Besides, most are women, because of their healthy habits, these older adults are less likely to develop chronic age-related diseases, such as high blood pressure, heart disease, cancer, and diabetes than their peers of the same age.

Siblings, as well as children (collectively called first-degree relatives) of long-term individuals, are more likely to stay healthy for longer and live up to ages older than their peers. People with centenary parents are less likely at age 70 to have age-related diseases that are common among the elderly. Centennial brothers and sisters generally have a long life and if they develop age-related diseases (such as hypertension, heart disease, cancer, or type 2 diabetes), these diseases appear later than in the general population. Longer lives tend to occur in families, suggesting that shared genetics, lifestyle, or both play an important role in determining longevity.

The study of longevity genes is a science in development. It is estimated that approximately 25 percent of the change in human life is determined by genetics, but which genes and how they contribute to longevity are not well known. Some of the common variations (called polymorphisms) associated with long periods of life are found in the APOE, FOXO3 and CETP genes but are not found in all individuals with exceptional longevity. Variations of multiple genes, some of which are not identified, are likely to work together to contribute to a long life.

Sequence studies of the entire genome of the Super centennial have identified the same genetic variants that increase the risk of disease in people who have an average life span. Supercentenarians also have many other newly identified genetic variants that are likely to promote longevity. Scientists speculate that during the first seven or eight decades, lifestyle is a stronger determinant of health and life than genetics. Eating well, avoiding drinking too much alcohol, avoiding tobacco, and staying physically active allows some people to reach a healthy old age; Therefore, genetics seems to play a progressively important role in keeping people healthy as they age since the 1980s and beyond. Many nonagenarians and centenarians can live independently and avoid age-related diseases until the last years of their lives.

Some of the genetic variants that contribute to a long life are involved in the maintenance and basic function of the body's cells. These cellular functions include the repair of DNA, maintenance of chromosomal ends (regions called telomeres), and cellular protection from damage caused by unstable oxygen-containing molecules (free radicals). Other genes associated with blood fat levels (lipids), inflammation and cardiovascular and immune systems contribute significantly to longevity, as they reduce the risk of heart disease (the leading cause of death in the elderly), stroke and insulin resistance

 In addition to studying antiquity in the United States, scientists also study a handful of communities in other parts of the world where people often live in their nineties and older: Okinawa (Japan), Ikaria (Greece) and Sardinia (Italy) These three regions are similar in the sense that they are relatively isolated from the general population in their countries, have a lower income, have little industrialization and tend to follow a traditional (non-Western) lifestyle. Unlike other ancient populations, the centenarians in Sardinia include a significant percentage of men. Researchers are investigating whether hormones, sex-specific genes or other factors can contribute to a longer life between men and women on this island.

CHAPTER ELEVEN

LONGEVITY DIET FOR ADULTS

Eat more vegetables, plus a little fish, limiting meals with fish to at most two or three per week. Select fish, crustaceans, and mollusks with a high omega-3, omega-6, and vitamin B12 content (salmon, anchovies, sardines, cod, sea bream, trout, clams, shrimp. Pay close attention to the quality of the fish, choosing only those who have low levels of mercury content.

If you are at the age with is below 65, moderate your protein intake to a minimum (0.31 to 0.36 grams per pound of body weight), which results to 40 to 47 grams of proteins per day for someone weighing 130 pounds, and 60 to 70 grams of protein per day for a person weighing 200 to 220 pounds. When you are over the age 65, you should slightly increase your protein intake but also increase the consumption of fish, eggs, white meat, and products derived from goats and sheep to preserve muscle mass. Eat beans, chickpeas, green peas, and other legumes as your major source of protein.

Minimize the level of saturated fats from animal and vegetable sources and sugar, and maximize good fats and complex carbs. Eat whole grains and high levels of vegetables (tomatoes, broccoli, carrots, legumes, etc.) with generous and adequate amounts of olive oil (3 tablespoons per day) and nuts (1 ounce per day).

Stick to a diet with a high level of vitamin and mineral content, supplemented with a multivitamin buffer every three to four days.

Select ingredients from those discussed in this book.

Based on your weight, age, and circumference of the abdomen will help you to decide whether to have two or three meals per day. Assuming that you are overweight or tend to gain weight with ease, consume two meals a day; breakfast and either lunch or dinner, as well as two low-sugar (less than 5 grams) snacks which are lesser than 100 cal each. If you are already at a moderate weight, you tend to lose weight easily or are over 65 and of moderate weight, eat three meals a day and one low-sugar snack, which can be less than three to five grams with fewer than 100 cal.

Confine all eating to within a 12 hours period; for example, start after 8 a.m. and end before 8 p.m. It is advisable not to eat anything within three to four hours of bedtime.

LONGEVITY DIET IN PREGNANCY

In pregnancy, it is important to pay particular attention to nutrition, not only for the baby in the womb but also for his or her future health as an adult.

It is a myth that pregnant women should "eat for two." Use the following table to calculate the correct weight gain according to BMI:

a. Underweight women (BMI less than 18.5): weight increase of 12.5-18 kg;

b. Women of normal weight (BMI 18.5-24.9): weight increase of 11.5-16 kg;

c. Overweight women (BMI greater than 25) or obese (BMI above 30): before getting pregnant, begin a personalized diet to lose weight.

Take precautions to avoid infections and avoid large fish that may contain mercury.

Do not eat raw meat, eggs or fish (even if packaged), unpasteurized milk and products — including soft cheeses like brie, Roquefort, gorgonzola, pâté, soft goat, sheep or cow's cheese, butter, cremes, ice cream, pre-packaged salads, sandwiches and street food such as hotdogs, or other pre-wall foods. Tofu, aged cheese like cheddar, Edam, Swiss, Gruyere, and parmesan, mozzarella, feta, ricotta, and spreadable cheeses are all safe choices.

Avoid high and long cooking temperatures, fried foods, and grilled meats.

Wash your hands frequently and carefully wash vegetables (best with a disinfectant), while avoiding salad and other raw vegetables.

Keep cooked and raw foods separate.

Fish that has been frozen rapidly (and at least for four days), smoked foods, and raw, salt-preserved fish eliminate the risk of infection and thus can be eaten, even if smoked products are best avoided.

Include in your diet two times a week "oily" or "high-fat" fish like salmon, trout or herring.

Vary your diet as much as possible, with foods rich in vitamins and minerals, and if necessary, take a daily vitamin that contains folic acid (at least 400 mcg a day).

In case of vomiting or constipation, modify your diet and eating habits.

Vegans and vegetarians should consume vitamin B12, iron, folic acid, omega 3, vitamin D, and calcium, in addition to following the general dietary recommendations.

Consult nutritionist periodically.

Limit foods containing caffeine, salt, sugar, soy, eggs and saturated and trans. fats

Avoid alcohol and do not smoke.

Maintain a right level of physical activity.

LONGEVITY DIET IN ADOLESCENTS

The Longevity Diet is a complete dietary program appropriate even for little ones. It contains all the nutrients children need: vegetable and animal proteins, carbohydrates, and fats.

Protein content should be regulated by age. Children should consume the following grams of protein, per kilo of body weight, each day:

- 1.3 grams up to 1 year old;

- 1 gram from 1 to 4 years old;

- 0.9 grams from 4 years and up.

For example, a 9-months-old baby who weighs 9 kg should consume 11.7 grams of protein a day; a toddler 3-years-old weighing 14 kg should consume 14 grams a day, and a child of 10 years old weighing 30 kg should consume approximately 27 grams a day.

Consume both vegetable-based proteins from legumes and nuts, and animal protein from fish (2-3 times a week, yet avoiding fish high in mercury), while eating less frequently red meat, white meat, and eggs (1 serving a week for each of these foods, and ideally organic).

Consume abundant quantities of carbohydrates with a low glycemic index (legumes and vegetables), thus reducing foods with high starch content (the 4Ps: "pasta", "pane" (bread), "pizza", "potatoes" + rice) and sugars (fruit, fruit juices, snacks, and sweetened carbonated beverages). However, to reduce does not mean cut out altogether, but rather consume minimal amounts.

Eat whole wheat foods with caution and other foods high in fiber like legumes if the child shows signs of intestinal discomfort. In such cases, consult with a pediatric gastroenterologist.

Reduce to the utmost minimum saturated, hydrogenated, and trans. Fats Limit salt and sugar. Still, sweets can be eaten in moderation, every so often, especially healthy ones made with fruit and dark chocolate.

Eat within a 12-hour period, e.g., begin with breakfast at 8 a.m and end with dinner at 8 p.m. This is especially important for children that are overweight and obese. Small exceptions can be made (i.e., 11 or 13-hour periods) if bodyweight is within the norm.

Meals and snacks must not exceed 4-5 a day.

Use a scale to keep track of weight and a flexible measuring tape to measure waist circumference. Take measurements with the following frequency:

Once a month for children of normal weight;

b. Once every two days for overweight, obese, and underweight children.

Eat more — not less. For children in general, and especially overweight kids, substitute high-starch foods like pasta, bread, rice, and potatoes with vegetables and legumes, which are rich in fiber and therefore fill you up faster. For example, take 50-60 grams of the starch-rich foods each day and substitute with 100 or more grams of carrots, broccoli, chickpeas, beans, etc.

Be somewhat flexible with the rules so that you find the right plan for each child, particularly with the help of a nutritionist. For example, if it makes a child happy, let him or her indulge in a can of soda and pizza once a week, and then make substitutions suggested at point 10 of this list.

Choose ingredients recommended in this book but give precedence to local, seasonal, and organic ingredients and those eaten by your ancestors — as much as possible.

Do at least one hour of exercise (sports) and an hour of walking a day.

CHAPTER TWELVE

58 WAYS TO LIVE A LONGER LIFE

1. Sing: Swedish researchers have discovered that singing has improved heart health. More research is being done at the University of California, San Francisco, to determine if singing can lead to a longer and healthier life.

2. For men, it is about marriage: according to The Longevity Project, men who married and remained so, probably lived more than 70 years, but less than a third of divorced men reached that age. Men who never married never survived those who divorced, but not those who remained married. Marital status made a small difference for women.

3. Work hard and be conscientious: Discovered by Project Longevity, people with conscientious personality traits and workers had a longer average life of two to three years, equivalent to a reduced risk of 20-30% death.

4. Eat berries: berries do not receive the "superfood miracle" label for nothing; The benefits of eating berries are practically too numerous to mention. Almost everyone will benefit from the consumption of berries, but here are the 11 tips for fat people to improve their health.

5.Always stay connected: people who have a social network, such as real-life friends, families or other communities, tend to live longer and healthier.

6. Put on your sneakers: and then run. You don't have to be a marathon runner to enjoy the benefits of running. The researchers found that runners lived on average three years longer than their non-runners and that running a minimum of 30 minutes to 59 minutes each week at a rate of fewer than 6 miles per hour offered the same health benefits of running periods Longer or faster.

7. Don't give up: A 13-year study found that among men and women who drank coffee, mortality rates decreased with the number of cups per day, up to six. The trend has been observed for deaths due to a variety of causes, including heart disease, respiratory disease, stroke as well as diabetes. Another survey of more than 1,600 people aged 90 and over found that those who drank moderate amounts of coffee (or alcohol) lived longer than those who abstained. For more information on how alcohol can be useful.

8. Be like Jean Calment: Who holds the world record for the duration of confirmed human life belongs, who lived for 122 years and 164 days. When asked what was the magic to his long life, he attributed it to a diet rich in olive oil, port wine, and two kilos of chocolate every week.

9. Take off your back: stop sitting so much! One study found that the session could be responsible for about

173,000 cases of cancer each year. Concentrating on the American population as a whole, another study which was concluded that if people remained seated less than three hours a day, on average, life expectancy would increase by two years. A team of doctors as well as researchers, also discovered that exchanging 30 minutes of sitting at high intensity can reduce a person's risk of premature death by 17%. Increase the intensity to moderate or vigorous exercise for 30 minutes and the risk decreases by 35%.

10. Help yourself for the right reasons: people who volunteer for altruistic reasons live longer than those who don't do charity or volunteer activities. (However, self-centered volunteers do not get the same benefits that prolong life!)

11. Don't worry, be happy: a Boston University study has linked optimism with long life. The researchers followed 71,173 women and men and found that the most optimistic people showed, on average, a lifespan of 11% to 15% more and were 50 to 70% more likely to reach 85 years compared to less optimistic groups. Another research done by the University of Texas discovered that those with a positive attitude were significantly less likely to become fragile than negative. Scientists have suggested that a positive outlook could affect health by altering the body's chemical balance.

12. Embrace your inner Grinch: this goes against expectations, but here it goes. According to data from a large 10-year survey, older Germans who were more pessimistic tended to live longer and healthier lives than their counterparts with a more positive outlook.

13. Eat like a Sicilian: When researchers began examining a significantly large group of centenarians on the island of Sicily, they discovered some things in common, particularly the fact that they all ate a diet rich in fruits, vegetables, and whole grains. and poor in red meat, refined carbohydrates and sweets.

14. Go to the Mediterranean in general: according to another study, about 30% of heart attacks, strokes and deaths from heart disease can be prevented in high-risk people assuming they switch to a Mediterranean diet. Possibly: nuts, olive oil, and wine, along with fresh fruits and vegetables, legumes, and fish;   Commercially produced biscuits and cakes should be avoided and dairy products and processed meats should be limited.

15. Add a pinch of turmeric: given all its vitality, it is not surprising that this bright orange spice is rich in antioxidants that fight disease. Turmeric is also proving to be a powerful anti-inflammatory.

16. Go for a walk: the benefits of a daily walk are many and include a significant reduction in the risk of developing type 2 diabetes, stroke, and dementia. But walk briskly.

17. Be a fast walker: how fast you can walk can indicate your longevity. because one study found that a 70-year-old man who walks 2.5 miles per hour compared to the same age that walks only 1 mile per hour should live eight years longer than the slowest man. If you are a woman, the difference is ten years! A 2019 study uncovered that people who walk faster are more likely to live longer, regardless of how much they are weighing.

 18. Eat less: You probably don't prefer hearing it, but if humans react in some way to a species of rhesus monkey in a study, the result is to reduce calories by 30% (keeping all the necessary ingredients for optimal health) in less diabetes, cancer, heart and brain diseases.

 19. Look at the vodka: this may not surprise anyone exactly: an in-depth study in Russia found that men who drank three or more half-liter vodka bottles per week were much more likely to die before reaching 55 years than those who reported having drunk less than one bottle per week. A quarter of Russian men die before age 55; many of those deaths are attributed to drinking.

 20. Stop smoking: we know you know, but anyway, we have to acknowledge it. According to the findings done by the centers for Disease Control and Prevention (CDC), smoking is the leading cause of preventable death in the United States, causing every five deaths every year.

 21. Eat your vegetables: vegetables are one of the best foods to eat regularly; They are rich in fiber and offer numerous vitamins, minerals, and herbal compounds that are believed to help protect the body from heart disease, diabetes and perhaps even cancer. Here are 15 to add to your diet.

22. Hugs: Research shows that contact with a loved one releases oxytocin, a stress-releasing hormone that helps reduce blood pressure. Lowering blood pressure means better heart health.

23. Laugh as often as possible: laughter dilates blood vessels by 22%, increasing blood flow and reducing blood pressure in the body circulatory system.

24. Eat broccoli: abundant with vitamin C, folic acid, and carotenoids, broccoli is rich in nutrients that protect your cells from free radical damage, improve immune system function and improve reproductive health.

25. Take a pet: research has found that people with pets tend to have lower blood pressure and are less likely to have hypertension than those without a pet.

26. Tight sleep: poor night-time sleep can lead to higher blood pressure, depression, weight gain, and cancer.

26. But then, wake up! assuming you sleep more than 9 hours a night. Studies show that sleeping more than 9 hours a night is related to an increased risk of heart disease, thinking problems and premature death.

27. Eat your vegetables: and sauté the meat. The American Dietetic Association found out that those who follow a properly planned vegetarian diet have a lower risk of developing heart disease; colorectal, ovarian and breast cancers; diabetes; the obesity; and hypertension

28. Plants: A growing number of studies have discovered the amazing benefits of the physical and mental health of gardening.

29. Drink hot chocolate: Yes, you heard correctly. Rejoice! By helping you think better about improving heart health, the antioxidants in hot chocolate are more concentrated than in many other sources, resulting in a lot of benefits to our health.

30. Savor sauerkraut: This has its uniqueness from its probiotic nature to its high vitamin content and its potential to fight cancer. Sauerkraut has a surprising range of health benefits.

31. Add ginger: Some studies have shown that, in addition to relieving muscle pain and helping with painful menstruation and migraines, ginger can eliminate inflammation and can even slow or kill cancer cells in the ovary and colon.

32. Beware of sports fanaticism: when the New York Giants beat the Patriots in the 2008 Super Bowl, the number of heart-related circulatory deaths in Massachusetts increased by 20% over the next eight days, which highlights the fact that deaths can increase or decrease in a region depending on how local teams are. Believe it or not, a heart attack is just one of the other health risks of being a sports fan.

33. Drink a drink: Even if it's not for everyone, a study from the University of Texas at Austin found that mortality rates were higher for those who never drank, lower for those who drank excessively, and lower for drinkers Moderates who enjoy one to three drinks per day.

34. Be happy: when examining data from 68,000 adults over ten years, one study found that the higher the level of depression or anxiety the participants experienced, the more likely they were to die during the period.

35. Skip the soda: studies show that drinking sugary drinks increases the risk of chronic diseases such as diabetes, heart disease, and cancer; One study found that drinking sugary drinks is related to 180,000 deaths a year worldwide.

36. Dodge smog: long-term exposure to air pollution is associated with an increased risk of premature death. In fact, studies have related 1 in 8 deaths worldwide with dirty air.

37. Eat dark chocolate: many studies agree that the effects of lowering blood pressure on dark chocolate consumption are useful in the prevention of cardiovascular issues.

38. Spend time with nature: When you spend a few hours in the forest, you breathe phytocides, active substances released by plants that seem to lower blood pressure and stress and strengthen the immune system.

39. Kick sugar: many experts claim that sugar cause obesity, diabetes, heart disease, and many other diseases that affect modern society.

40. Add honey: replacing refined sugar with genuine honey can offer many health benefits.

41. Choose a recreational sport: skating, bowling, fencing, volleyball? Just some of the fun activities that offer a wide range of health benefits. Ping pong has also improved motor functions and long-term memory functions.

42. Keep calm and continue. And do not be angry. Harvard research has found that in the two hours after an outbreak of rabies, a person's risk of heart attack has increased by almost five times and the risk of stroke has increased more than three times.

43. Drinking tea: from anti-cancer properties to reducing the risk of coronary heart disease and reducing the risk of blood clots and strokes, tea is a true draft horse in the health department.

44. Eat wild salmon: Eating wild salmon provides us with one of the richest sources of omega-3 fats out there, which can help reduce triglycerides, increase HDL ("good") cholesterol levels and help reduce inflammation in the body.

45. Transmit burned food: evidence continues to state that chemical acrylamide, present in burned food, can cause cancer.

46. Beware of the deadly apple: as well as other poisonous foods we normally consume.

47. Reduce your TV screen time: a large Australian study found that although the participants did an average of 30-45 minutes of daily exercise, their risk of death from cardiovascular disease increased by 18% per hour per day watching television.

48. Eat oatmeal for breakfast: for many reasons, and here are 12 ways to do it.

49. Dance! It is believed that physical activity reduces the risk of Alzheimer's by 50%. And one study found that frequent dancing reduces the risk of developing dementia by an incredible 76%, more than any other physical or cognitive activity.

50. Give us: from the department "oh, baby": sex is good for increasing immunity and heart health.

51. Eliminate the habit of instant noodles? Can be. One study discovered that eating instant noodles two or more times a week was associated with cardiometabolic syndrome, which increases the likelihood of a person developing heart disease and other conditions, such as diabetes and stroke.

52. Do not avoid garlic: studies indicate that garlic's active ingredient can prevent atherosclerosis and coronary blockage, reduce cholesterol, reduce blood clot formation, regulate blood sugar, and prevent cancer.

53. Go for a walk after eating: according to one study, walking and training in light resistance one hour after eating a high-fat meal reduces the increase in triglycerides (blood fats that may increase the risk of heart disease) normally observed after the consumption of this type of food.

54. Nut snack: Nuts of all types have many healthy fats and heart proteins, two components that keep blood sugar stable by decreasing the rate at which your body absorbs carbohydrates. Walnuts also contain monounsaturated fats and, in some cases, omega-3s, which improve cholesterol and triglyceride levels.

55. Take an aspirin: If you previously had a heart attack or stroke, or if you have diabetes, taking aspirin every day can prolong your life.

56. Consume pumpkin seeds: do not let those good seeds be wasted; They are small nutrient feeders.

57. Take care of your teeth: periodontal disease could be directly related to systemic inflammation and cardiovascular risk. According to the American Academy of Periodontics, people with gum disease are twice as likely to have heart disease.

58. Exercise: I knew we should have said it, and this is just one example of why: time reports that an in-depth study found that even only 15 minutes of moderate exercise per day was associated with a three-year increase in expectation. Of life compared to those who have not exercised. And people who normally exercised for 30 minutes a day added four more years to their life expectancy.

CHAPTER THIRTEEN

THE SECRETS OF STAYING YOUNG AND BEAUTIFUL

Aging is a natural and inevitable process. However, aging gracefully does not have to mean sitting down and enjoying the trip without trying to delay it. Numerous things are out there that you can perform to maintain your youthful appearance and beauty for as long as possible, without being unpleasant. So, if you're ready, here are some beauty and anti-aging secrets you should know, ranging from daily routine tricks to more serious efforts.

Protect your skin from the sun: The sun can be a friend of your skin because it provides you with much-needed vitamin D. However if you overexpose your skin to the sun and especially if it occurs when the sun is most active, it can significantly accelerate the aging process. So how do you protect your skin from this bad influence? There are several ways. First and foremost, and most importantly, apply sunscreen every time you go out (yes, even during winter). Even sunglasses are useful, but for full-face coverage and to avoid hyperpigmentation, make hats part of your outerwear.

Skincare for your skin type: Products of all skin types are generally absurd because we all expect different effects of each product. The solution would be to have a beautician who prepares creams and lotions for your unique skin, but as it is almost impossible, you can always find a line of products that matches your skin type (for example, oily, dry, normal).

A seasonal routine: You do not wear the same clothes during summer and winter, so why should you use the same skincare products in both seasons? The cold causes cracks, irritation, and cracks in the skin, while the heat requires additional protection against sunburn. Hydration is essential for each season, but during the winter and fall months, it is more important than ever. Also, an additional tip for each season: don't forget your neck and neckline when you take care of your face.

Regenerating facial treatments: Despite all the products for skincare and protection, sometimes the years take its toll and you need some extra help to recover the previous shine of your skin. Fortunately, today there are dozens of effective anti-aging treatments that you can try, such as anti-wrinkle injections, dermal fillers, platelet-rich plasma, medical needles for the skin, stretching of threads and stretching of the eyelid skin.

Keep your body fit: A healthy diet and exercise are crucial not only to keep you fit and make your clothes more suitable, but they can also shave you years after your age and improve your health to the point where you will look much younger than you really are. It also keeps the skin shiny, improves posture and flexibility, helps you sleep better, and slows aging.

Ask for help: Sometimes, exercise is not enough for your body to have the shape you want, and that's fine. Not everyone can look like the best models. However, there are ways to get rid of persistent abdominal fat and look much better. If you are dealing with a slight surplus in that area, you can try non-invasive procedures, such as co-culture, and if you have more problem areas with more than a slight surplus, there are many sensational procedures. While reading this, 3D liposuction in Perth and other Australian cities is becoming one of the most popular ways to achieve an athletic and sensual body shape with minimal effort.

Take care of your appearance: Of course, beauty is not all about skin, and the dress and hair are not women, but they can be used to make you look more beautiful and young. For example, shorter hairstyles or well-fed shiny hair can be instant rejuvenators. Also, dressing for your figure is very important. It should not be limited to dark and changing color tones; Green, yellow, and red can look good regardless of their age and make it look a couple of years younger.

Finally, put a smile on that face: there is no better way to look young than to feel young. Surround yourself with positive, friendly, and fun people and be happy: that's all.

HOW CAN YOU STAY YOUNG AND HEALTHY?

Being involved in the daily routine of life can leave you angry, stressed and worried about many things. Worries can show on your face and when that occurs, stress will begin to appear on your face as wrinkles and facial lines. If you want to prepare mentally and physically for all life experiences, let go of jumbled thoughts, continue with the flow of life and understand that this is the best way to stay young.

Age-related changes in the body:

The face begins to show the age lines in middle age and people want to keep their appearance young and fresh forever.

In addition to the appearance, mood swings and hormonal changes begin to take control and the body shape is disturbed.

Bones weaken, energy levels decrease, weight increases, fatigue takes over, and sexual dysfunction arises with increasing age. The only thought that begins to create problems is how to stay young looking for 40 years.

How can you keep your body healthy and face the young?

A healthy body reflects a radiant face and young skin. People often wonder about keeping their skin young. How to prevent aging? Staying beautiful or young is not the result of treatments; It requires great efforts and can only be achieved by applying a natural skincare treatment.

With age, the skin's natural collagen begins to run out. Collagen supplementation can work wonders on the skin because empty spaces fill up. The lines are stretched and removed.

How to stay healthy? This is a question that bothers many people. The best way to stay beautiful and young is to clean the skin and ingest many vitamins and nutrients from the diet. Eat healthily, stay healthy.

Free yourself from stress by doing meditation, yoga or following your favorite hobbies and you won't have to ask yourself. "How to keep your skin young?". Doing activities that interest you will make you happy and the stress lines will soon begin to dissipate. Stressed people begin to gain weight and age faster. Stress leads to a disruption in the production of hormones and can accelerate the aging process. So try to find ways to relax so you can always stay young and beautiful.

Detoxification of the body and skin is essential. That includes cleansing the skin and body. Regularly stocking fresh fruits and vegetables can provide a healthy glow to dry, flaccid skin. Fruits, as well as vegetables, contain antioxidants, minerals, and vitamins that aid in keeping the body young and fresh.

The modern beauty industry has developed natural creams for skincare after much research. These applications contain minerals and ingredients that spoil the skin from the depths. A regular application will help you stay young and beautiful.

Regular exercise helps secrete happy hormones and endorphins. Blood circulation greatly improves and high energy levels improve moods, thereby relieving stress when going to the gym or taking a long and rejuvenating walk.

No swollen eye and a gloriously lit face are the results of a long and restful night. People who lie down and sleep well have high energy levels and better health. In a night of deep sleep, the pituitary gland begins to function efficiently. In the first phase of a proper deep sleep, it secretes growth hormones in adequate amounts. If sleep is disturbed or inappropriate, the secretion of the pituitary gland becomes irregular. This hormonal imbalance accelerates the aging process.

Control your emotional disorder positively so you can avoid any kind of coercive situation in life. Staying calm and serene will help you maintain the same behavior in all cases. Keep stressful breaks at bay and rely on fun and humor to deal with difficulties. You will notice that your face always remains bright and radiant.

Diet and nutrition: data are vital to staying young along with persistence

Staying young and in good shape forever was the burning desire of everyone in today's modern and fast world. This desire has its roots in the distant past of humanity, is there today and will persist forever until there are human beings. Ancient herbs and medicinal therapies have the same importance as those of modern drugs and modern sciences in the perseverance of this man's desire.

Diet and nutrition determine the success or otherwise in staying young and fit. The fact that food is very different from its nutritional value is at the center of the idea. What you eat and how much you eat decides your health and age limit. Once young age ends, it is very difficult to stay young and fit, since nature must fulfill its duties. It is beyond man's reach to prevent nature from carrying out its tasks, but man can prolong the aging process with the help of correct information and constant efforts.

Nutrition facts and diet information are available in abundance today. Diet programs and programs, diet recipes, and nutritional values are there to help a man stay young and fit. The only thing is that you must study carefully and choose between the available dietary data if you want to prolong the aging process and stay healthy. Only a weight loss pill or simply a weight loss program will not help the man in this regard.

Regular exercise is mandatory and you cannot succeed if you really want to stay young and fit. Therefore, rest depends entirely on eating habits and nutritional values of food intake to satisfy that burning and passionate desire of man. Whoever abides by the laws of nature, nature becomes generous with him.

STAY YOUNG AND HEALTHY

We all love to stay young and healthy for a long time and yet we don't have a potion for this. It is not necessary to have a potion. Some regulations in our lives can limit the aging process and diseases. We will stay fit even in the sixth and seventh decades of our lives. But the fact is that we are going to grow old, that's for sure. We will discuss here how we can slow down the process.

First, we must have a positive mental attitude. Yes, attitude plays a vital role in the quest to stay younger. Many of us are skeptical or really surprised to know this truth. You may wonder if we need to remain young forever. The great anti-aging secret is that you could have better health accompanied by a positive attitude and the power of positive thinking.

The role of the exercise continues. Challenging your body through different exercise programs will bring the benefit of staying disease-free and having a high mental level. Once you have started exercising, you will automatically start taking nutritious foods. This is probably one of the key aspects of staying young and healthy for a long time. The antioxidants of a balanced diet will keep free radicals at bay, which are the main culprits of premature aging. Enough antioxidants in your body will continually create a well-maintained immune system that will also keep your body safe from disease.

Stress is another powerful inducer of the aging process. Being stress-free is not entirely possible, but we can do something that releases stress from our minds. Relaxation techniques involve yoga and meditation. Try to be calm, cool and collected in any situation. Smiling even in very uncomfortable situations will help reduce stress. In addition, smiling will tone the face and the person will look much younger. The neurotransmitters released during the smile have a beneficial effect on the aging process.

Peradventure, one of the most recognizable aspects of the younger aspect is healthy skin. The aging process and pollution take its toll and the skin becomes wrinkled and shiny. There are several herbal medicines and cosmetic products available in the market that can revitalize the skin and stop the formation of wrinkles. But they are almost always very publicized and they are doing worse. You should buy a product that suits your skin type and that has enough customer testimonials to prove your request.

The motivation to be young and healthy is also important. We should have a few minutes for ourselves and discuss the benefits of staying healthy for a long time. Then only we can gather the energy and ambition to reach them. It is always better to be optimistic about those wonderful things that the future has saved us.

Set yourself a set of goals and join them one by one. In this way, your attention to stay young and healthy will not be lost and the road will be easier to follow.

HOW TO GET SUPER HEALTH: STAY YOUNG AND ACTIVE

Vitamin A, beta-carotene, vitamin E, and selenium are food supplements that work together as an excellent rejuvenator, preventing a large number of diseases and diseases, such as those derived from the natural aging process. They also neutralize the "free radicals" that cause these problems.

Beta carotene is a provitamin that is converted into vitamin A through a process that occurs in the liver and intestinal walls. When this vitamin is taken with vitamin E and selenium, its healing and nutritional qualities greatly improve.

Beta carotene or vitamin A helps prevent night blindness. From here comes the saying, "Eat carrots so you can see at night." Beta carotene is essential to produce a substance called visual violet that you need to be able to see better at night or in very little night.

The lack of beta-carotene also causes skin disorders, causes dryness in the mucous membranes of the nose, lungs, and mouth or stimulates the production of acne.

Beta-carotene helps prevent problems caused by excessive contamination, and it also helps delay the production of ulcers and prevent the formation of cancerous tumors. In addition, it has been discovered that this vitamin is important in the formation of bones and teeth. It acts as a molecular oxidizing agent that helps protect cells from a variety of diseases such as cancer.

Vitamin E is another very important element to prevent tissue wear, and it is also called tocopherol, this vitamin that is stored in the liver, in adipose tissues, in the heart, in muscles, in the testicles, in the uterus, in the blood and in the adrenal and pituitary glands. It dilates blood vessels, is a coagulant and improves circulation, strengthens capillary walls, helps fertility and male potency, protects the lungs, prevents and dissolves blood clots, maintains muscles and nerves.

Selenium combined with vitamins E and A strongly increases the activity of these vitamins. The same happens when mixed with magnesium.

Vitamin E also helps you stay young by slowing the aging process that occurs due to oxidation, neutralizes free radicals and also supplies oxygen to the body, giving it a stronger resistance. It also protects the lungs from contamination, acts together with vitamin A, dissolves blood clots and relieves fatigue and prevents the formation of heavy scar tissue, accelerates the healing of burns and prevents spontaneous abortions, also relieves cramps in the legs, prevents the destruction of red blood cells, muscle degeneration, anaemia and disorders of the reproductive system, acts as a prevention against cancer and cardiovascular problems, in addition to helping improve circulation, repair tissues and is of great It helps in the treatment of high blood pressure.

SEVEN FOODS TO AVOID STAYING YOUNG

What does food have to do with young people? Why are we discussing diets? Because you are what you eat and beauty, as well as youth, are the natural reflection of healthier living and well-being, and health is closely linked to what we eat. Look. No matter how much we can control our temperament, attitude, and mentality, we need to eat correctly to stay healthy. There is no doubt or argument about this.

For most of us, eating is one of the most satisfying things we do in everyday life. It is one of the greatest sources of pleasure. Instead, eating often has become one of our favorite hobbies. Therefore, we will definitely need to learn to eat well to stay healthy and young.

Below are some daily foods to prevent them from damaging our health if they are taken in excess. In most cases, I will use the word healthy instead of young.

1. Dairy products

Accepting too much can cause heart problems. Dairy products are mucous and difficult to digest. If they eat, a better option would be to accompany them with salad. Take care of your consumption.

2. Processed foods

Overeating processed and preserved food is harmful to our health. First, they contain hidden sugar, extra salt, flavor enhancer, food conditioner, and other additives that contribute to health problems. Second, harmful preservatives are added to make food "fresh" for longer. Third, it has no nutritional value, even though they were good foods before canning because processing brought most of the nutrients from nutrient-rich foods.

3. Genetically modified foods (GMO)

Genetic engineering is said to be a radical new technology that breaks the fundamental genetic barriers not only between species but also between humans, animals and plants in an unnatural way. A good reason to worry is that these laboratory-created foods that are not safe for human consumption. There is no specific way to differentiate between GM, natural and organic potatoes, soy, corn or tomatoes, etc. They have been genetically modified. The only way to avoid these GM foods is to eat and buy organic foods, if possible. If you plan to grow and produce your own food, buy only organic seeds.

4. Refined food

White flour, white rice and white sugar are processed foods. They are made by stripping cereals and canes of all available natural nutrients: fiber, vitamins and minerals to give them a relatively clean and white color. They become impoverished and transformed "dead" foods that often contribute to constipation and other digestive and health problems. Since all nutrients are virtually eliminated, the most refined foods should be enriched with synthetic vitamins and minerals. But keep in your inner thought that our body cannot process chemical nutrients.

5. Hydrogenated / partially hydrogenated

Hydrogenation is the process of artificially converting natural liquid oil (vegetable oil) into solid form at room temperature, such as margarine, nut butter, cookies, cookies, and powdered drinks, etc. From this hydrogenation process, harmful trans-fatty acids are created to cause blood clots, heart problems, cancer, and other degenerative diseases. Read the labels and avoid anything hydrogenated. And don't be fooled by the tag which generally says "partially hydrogenated oil," partially hydrogenated oil is worse than fully hydrogenated oil!

6. microwave food

According to a research book published by Dr. Hans Ulrich Hertel and a professor at the University of Lausanne, foods cooked in microwave ovens could present a greater health risk than foods cooked by conventional means. A microwave oven breaks down and the molecular structure of food changes through the radiation process. Microwave cooking creates carcinogens and causes a significant reduction in the nutritional value of food.

7. meat

Eating meat itself is not healthy. The study of the human digestive system has shown that it is not designed to eat meat from the beginning. Some meats, such as beef, take approximately 72 hours to digest completely. Therefore, if you eat meat at each meal, you would still digest the food you ate for breakfast the other day while consuming another round again.

A vegetarian diet is good because it eliminates the problem of indigestion due to an inadequate association of food that often leads to the fermentation and breakdown of food in the stomach. More importantly, the nutrients needed to rejuvenate and replenish our cells are destroyed in the process of decomposition and fermentation, often in the case of the meat-eater. That is one of the many reasons by which most people today look older than their real age; dietary diets and food cycles generally lead to premature aging and disease.

If you want to stay young and live a healthy life, minimize the intake of the aforementioned foods: dairy products, processed foods, refined foods, microwaves, and GM foods, hydrogenated oil, and meat. Replace meat with healthier alternatives such as tofu. Turn vegetables into your daily business. Let the meat be the accompaniment and not the main course. Go for fresh fruits, vegetables, nuts, seeds, fresh and ripe for health and youth.

CONCLUSION

Well, we may not know for sure what the future of human health and longevity will be, but we can assume and predict it. It is known that high blood pressure increases the risk of heart disease, stroke and kidney failure, but only a few studies have examined how blood pressure affects longevity. Other things like having green trees in the neighborhood, exposing our body to sun, are linked to longevity. Deep sleep is probably the most important secret of longevity. Another secret is we should take many antioxidants in high doses – I believe that researchers' efforts could significantly improve the future of human health and longevity, as well as advances in antioxidant and anti-aging medicine.